THE DARK THREADS

THE DARK THREADS

A Psychiatric Survivor's Story

Jean Davison

Published by Accent Press Ltd – 2009

ISBN 9781906373597

Printed and bound in the UK by CPI Bookmarque

Cover Design by The Design House

To Ian

Grateful acknowledgement is made to the following for permission to reproduce copyright material:

'Time-bomb' poem. Reproduced by kind permission of the author, Professor Valerie Walkerdine.

Nineteen Eighty-Four by George Orwell (Copyright © George Orwell, 1949) by permission of Bill Hamilton as the Literary Executor of the Estate of the late Sonia Brownell Orwell and Secker & Warburg Ltd.

Extract from 'Aftermath' poem. By kind permission of the author, Leonard Roy Frank.

Two lines of 'Stings' from *Collected Poems* by Sylvia Plath. Reproduced by permission of Faber and Faber Ltd.

Quotation from *To Kill a Mockingbird* by Harper Lee, published by William Heinemann Ltd. Reprinted by permission of The Random House Group Ltd.

Extract from 'The Weaver' poem. By kind permission of E Sue Wagner and family of the late Benjamin Malachi Franklin.

AUTHOR'S NOTE

The Dark Threads is an autobiographical account of 'breakdown' and psychiatric treatment. I have used some of the techniques of writing fiction (dialogue, imagery, fictitious names/identifying details) to protect people's privacy and also to facilitate self-expression. The names of medical professionals have been changed. Instead of using my maiden name I have used my married surname of Davison throughout the book (although my actual case notes were, of course, in my maiden name). In some instances I've fleshed out half-remembered scenes with invented minor details, such as the colour of a bedspread, the weather, an ink stain on a desk. But I have not, to my knowledge, distorted the substance of the true story.

No more, I will accept no more
                    be sorry no more
be quiet no more
They will have to hear my story
and they will not dare to say it
                    made me mad
Of course it made me mad
After all they pathologised
                    my history
No more, no more
my shouts today will be
                    so loud
My tears drops of pure fire
you will no longer take away
                    my past
for today I take my life
into these two hands

I am a time-bomb
and I have started ticking

                    Valerie Walkerdine

PROLOGUE

'WE ARE IN GRAVE danger!' a voice insists.

I can hear the words, but from somewhere distant. I keep floating away. A blurred, drugged sensation. Sounds of moaning. Stench of vomit and urine. I feel the hardness of the mattress, the roughness of the blanket. I am trying to focus my eyes on a ghostly figure beside my bed, but semi-darkness encircles me.

I remember hearing screams. I grip the blanket. What else do I remember? My befuddled brain throws up a vague recollection of being held down firmly and suffocating blackness. Nothing makes sense. Exorcism? Purgation? Trials and torture? But where are the witches? We don't burn witches any more. We don't believe in witches now. The Dark Ages are gone but, oh, it is not safe here. There is a grey mist about me; someone keeps warning of grave danger; and my head hurts so badly. I have had a very strange dream, a terrible nightmare. Am I awake or am I still dreaming?

After a half-hearted attempt to sit up I succumb to the seduction of the pillow to rest my aching head. This is not the same as an ordinary headache, more like the soreness of a nasty bump. But not a surface lump. It is somewhere inside my head; this soreness, this dull, throbbing pain.

My eyes follow the white-clad figure. It is not a ghost but a nurse. She is moving to the next bed. There on the bed, a thin, straggly-haired woman is stretching her arms towards me and warning of danger.

'We are in grave danger!' She is even more insistent. Her voice is shaky and hoarse.

I am aware now that my bed is in a row of beds. One woman is sitting on the edge of her bed vomiting into a bowl. Some are moaning, others lying quiet and still.

Where am I? What day is it? Who are these people? And who am I? Please don't give me a number or a label or a curious sidelong glance. Tell me my name.

Creeping tentacles of fear spread over my body, reminding me of waiting – that long anxiety-filled stretch of waiting. Before ECT. That's it! We're waiting for electric shock treatment. The nurse is standing near my bed. It must be my turn. Ripples of apprehension run from my stomach to my throat, then settle into a tight knot of fear somewhere inside my chest. Perhaps if I tell her I feel ill I'll be able to get out of it. God knows it isn't a lie.

'Can I be excused ECT today?' I am begging her. 'I've a bad headache.'

The nurse laughs loudly as if it is all a huge joke. 'Excused ECT? You've *had* ECT.'

'Have I?' I say, bewildered. 'But I don't remember.'

I feel as if half my brain has been bombed out but, oh, what a relief to know it is all over. At least for today.

'Be a good girl and get up now, then you can have a nice cup of tea.' The nurse is beaming pleasantly. Meekly I obey. Just like a good girl.

I am handed a cardboard container full of warm, muddy-looking liquid, which I suppose must be the nice cup of tea. It tastes foul.

'Don't drink it! They're trying to poison us!' a woman in a hospital dressing-gown whispers in my ear as she shuffles past.

Still in a trance, I survey my fellow sufferers. We're a mixed bunch. Some look as if they would give the devil himself a fright but most seem just lost, confused and so very vulnerable. 'Where are my teeth?' 'Where are my glasses?' 'Oh, the pain, I can't stand the pain.' 'I'll sue you all for this, you fucking bastards!'

As I listen to the other patients and watch them wandering around in a daze, I find it hard to believe it's real. Aren't these people mentally ill? But not me too? No, no, it must be a bad dream. Or there must have been a dreadful mistake. I shouldn't be here; a part of my mind is weeping and protesting against the horror and humiliation of it all. I'm losing my powers of reasoning and my self-respect. I've got to get out of here. I've got to get the hell out of here. Before it's too late.

But is it already too late? I have been violated at a deeper level than words can say. How can I ever be the same again?

Looking back through the drugged haze and post-ECT fog it seems strange to think that, only a fortnight earlier, I was walking through the park on my way to that first appointment at the outpatient clinic. I had never seen a psychiatrist, never even heard of ECT as I dawdled along, crunching underfoot the autumn leaves, those lovely golds and reds and russet browns which swirled about and decked the tree-lined path near the pond. Here I sat on a bench for a while, savouring the scene. It was turning cold but the pond was not yet frozen. The leaves were falling but the trees were not yet bare. Squirrels still darted about now and then, birds still sang and the ground was not yet shrouded in snow. But winter was fast approaching. Soon all would be changed.

Shouldn't there have been some kind of ritual, some rite of passage, to mark such a sudden and awesome transformation? One day I was living in a teenage world of discos, pop songs, dating, giggles with female friends, religious angst and worries about pimples. The next day I was in a nightmare world of drugs, ECT, humiliation and long, bleak corridors leading me far from home. And the only connecting thread, it seemed, was when I had calmly, and I thought sensibly, decided to see a psychiatrist and then agreed to be hospitalised.

How can this be? Have I forgotten something that might explain it all? If I begin by following that connecting thread, will it lead me to answers?

I am still trying to sort out my thoughts when the nurse tells us that an ambulance is waiting to take us back to our wards. How could I have been stupid enough to let my life get into such a mess? And how am I ever going to get myself out of it? I stumble into the ambulance feeling dizzy and disorientated.

The ambulance is bumping across the broken tarmac. In the far corner the hoarse voice keeps on saying, 'We are in grave danger!' I am sitting wedged between two plump, dressing-gown-clad patients with vacant, staring eyes. I am thinking about the God I don't believe in, my need of 'Him' accentuated by sheer desperation. Dear God in heaven. Friend of my childhood. Comforter and Guide. Where, oh where are You now?

PART ONE

A GOOD GIRL

Power is in inflicting pain and humiliation.
Power is in tearing human minds to pieces and putting them together again in new shapes of your own choosing.

George Orwell, *Nineteen Eighty-Four*

CHAPTER ONE

WE WERE AT BUTLINS, Skegness, in the August of 1968, my
friend Mandy and me. Two weeks with no boring lists to type
or envelopes to stick. Two weeks of sun, sand, sea and
boyfriends galore. Lots of kissing, petting, dancing, laughter
and ... and, all the time, the thoughts and feelings that had
plagued me for so long. Who am I? What am I? What to do?
How to be?

The jukebox in the disco played loudly while we, wearing
mini-skirts the size of napkins, danced the night away with two
handsome security guards, stopping now and then to kiss, and
to drink all the port and lemons they bought for us. We giggled
and clowned about all the way back to our chalet, locked the
lads out, and collapsed onto our beds, heads spinning. Still
chuckling, we prattled on about what a great time we were
having, what fun things we'd do tomorrow, and then on to the
bigger things such as how to put the world to rights. Teenage
life in the sixties. Who could wish for anything more?

We went to bed, then read for a while. I can't go on like
this, I told myself as I lay in my top bunk silently crying, a
magazine covering my face. Mandy was lying in bed beneath
me reading her magazine. She thought I was still reading mine,
but, in the middle of a girl-meets-boy romance, I'd started to
cry. It was nothing to do with the paper-thin girl in the shallow,
meaningless story. It was to do with me and my shallow,
meaningless life.

''Night, Jean,' Mandy murmured sleepily.

'Hang on, Mandy, don't put the light out yet. I've just got
me diary to write.'

It all came out in my diary: a place where I could be totally honest. 'I'm so terribly depressed,' I wrote. 'I'm eighteen and should be enjoying myself. It's not normal to be so sad and confused about life all of the time ... I've got to do something sensible about it.'

I decided that doing 'something sensible about it' meant that when I got back from Skegness I'd see a doctor.

Even so, I put this off until November, perhaps hoping I might yet manage to sort things out by myself. Came November with its fog and rain, and me still as adrift as a cork in the sea, I visited my doctor.

I first went to see Dr Russo on the pretext that I wanted some sleeping tablets, although what I really wanted was to talk. I thought asking for these would help me by providing me with an easier starting point. But ten minutes later, I left his surgery with a prescription for a small supply of sleeping tablets and the comment that I shouldn't need them at my age.

A few days later, my friend Jackie told me that she was at a low ebb, too. We both decided to visit our respective GPs, and so I tried again to talk to him.

'The beliefs of the church are disproved by science,' Dr Russo said when I tried to tell him about my confusion with religion.

With Dr Russo, I found myself defending the very beliefs which, in front of Pastor West and my family, I'd been so ardently rejecting. Yet beneath my rebellious onslaught against religion, there had been a challenge and an appeal to Pastor West: always, a silent plea for him to convince me that I was wrong.

When Jackie and I next met she told me that her GP had said she was suffering with nervous anxiety. We compared our bottles of tranquillisers, which we both found made us drowsy and impeded our concentration at work. I went back to Dr Russo and told him I felt worse than ever. He increased the dosage.

I couldn't see the point in taking tablets that made me too

tired to talk or do anything. There was so much inside me that needed to come out. I wanted to be understood. I *needed* to talk. It occurred to me that a psychiatrist might be more helpful than an overworked GP.

'What? You're going to ask Dr Russo if you can see a psychiatrist?' said my mother. 'What on earth for? There's nowt up with you.'

'Listen, Mum,' I began, though listening was something she never seemed to do. She always looked pale and exhausted; perhaps her job as a bus conductress was too tiring for her. 'I need someone to talk to and maybe a psychiatrist could help. I mean they're trained to understand people and –'

'You don't need a psychiatrist,' Mum said. 'You ought to go back to church.'

When I asked Dr Russo if I could see a psychiatrist he wrote out a medical certificate with the diagnosis 'acute depression' and said, 'Yes, I suppose we could try that, if you like.'

So that was it. If I'd known how easy it would be for me to see a psychiatrist I would probably have asked to see one a few years earlier. Between the ages of thirteen and fifteen I'd gained my knowledge of psychiatrists from *The Human Jungle*, my favourite TV programme at the time. Young and impressionable, I'd seen the psychiatrist Dr Corder, played by the actor Herbert Lom, as a wise, caring person who could help people with their problems. How wonderful it would be to have someone like that to talk to, someone who would take the time to really listen to me, and understand. It's embarrassing to admit it now but I'm sure *The Human Jungle* had something to do with my decision to ask to see a psychiatrist.

And so, on a crisp autumn day in 1968, I was fidgeting on a hard chair in the crowded outpatients department of St Luke's Hospital waiting to see Dr Sugden. I was surprised by the apparent normality of the others in the waiting area. But I looked ordinary too, didn't I?

Trying to ignore my butterflies I picked up a magazine and flicked through the pages. What if he didn't take me seriously? I had a boyfriend, female friends, an active social life, which might make it seem that my shyness wasn't such a problem. When boys chatted me up I could reciprocate. I'd had several boyfriends and I can't have seemed shy when laughing and chatting with them.

However, shyness did still keep me subdued in my office job at Lee's, and it had been an enormous problem before that in my first job at the Fisk Television factory. And at Rossfields, my last school, oh, God, I'd been crippled by shyness there.

And would this psychiatrist be able to understand my difficulties in coming to terms with the loss of my religious beliefs, about life seeming empty and meaningless, and those hard to explain 'What am I?' feelings? Perhaps he would try to impress upon me all that I ought to be thankful for. Or perhaps, like Pastor West, he would speak about that difficult transition period from adolescence to adulthood. Perhaps he would say there was nothing wrong with me and, horror of horrors, that I must go back to work tomorrow. I had no idea that this was the last thing I need have feared. Or that there would come a day when I would wish that he had.

When I was called into the consulting room my stomach was still churning. Dr Sugden was a frail, elderly man with metal-framed glasses, which slid down his nose every time he bent his head forward. It was hard to imagine that he could have much understanding of teenagers. But I tried not to judge on the basis of first impressions.

I shifted about on my seat. The pills prescribed by Dr Russo were making me feel too tired to want to talk but I tried to explain things. I even told him about the strange 'dream feeling' I used to get when I was a schoolgirl at Rossfields, and he seemed particularly interested in that, despite my admission that I only got it now when I'd been drinking. He scribbled on his notepad and kept saying 'I see', but I wasn't at all sure that he did.

For so long I'd been wanting the opportunity to have a good talk, but now all I could think of saying had come out in a few minutes and sounded like nothing much. I felt embarrassed for wasting his time.

'I'm scared. I'm scared I'm going insane,' I said. Shyness made my voice shaky, adding to the drama of this statement.

'Do you sometimes feel like killing yourself?' he asked.

I didn't, but would a straight 'No' make him underestimate how bad I felt? I paused for a while, then replied, 'I know that wouldn't be the right thing to do.'

'I see. And are you happy at home?'

Another pause. I'd told Mum I would talk about me, not my family. In any case, I was aware that many teenagers came from worse homes than mine.

'I feel as if I'm different from me family,' I said. 'And me brother gets on me nerves.' I hung my head guiltily. Sorry, Mum, but I need to talk.

'How old is your brother?'

'Twenty-two.'

'You don't feel able to talk to him about your problems?'

'Brian? Good heavens, no. I can't talk to him about owt.'

'What's his occupation?'

'He's a bus conductor. Like me mum and dad.' I gave a nervous smile. 'A family of bus conductors. Except me. I'm a typist at Lee's, an electrical firm.'

'You say your brother gets on your nerves,' he said, adjusting his hearing aid. 'What does he do?'

'All kinds of things,' I said uneasily.

'What things?'

'Well, he talks daft and bangs and taps and ... and he makes silly noises.'

'Silly noises? What are these silly noises like?'

'Noises like animals,' I said.

'Give me an example to show me what you mean.'

God, this was difficult. I decided to demonstrate Brian's cow noises which he'd been treating me to outside my bedroom door in the early hours of that very morning.

'OK, that's enough of that,' Dr Sugden said, waving his hand on my third 'Mooo-ooo!'

'I can't stop thinking about religion,' I said quickly, trying

11

to get away from the embarrassing subject of my family. 'I used to go to church but I got confused with some of their beliefs. I mean, things such as God sending people to hell to suffer for eternity. I can't believe in things like that, so I stopped going. But when I lost me religious beliefs, everything began to seem pointless.'

'Your life seems pointless?'

'Yes, and I'm confused all the time. I don't even know how to decide what's right and wrong.'

I was thinking that, although, for many of my generation, the pill had rendered outdated the idea of saving virginity for marriage, my decision not to sleep with boyfriends had been anchored in my Christian beliefs. Not even smooth-talking Steve, the most handsome of my previous boyfriends, had been able to persuade me, despite the physical attraction between us. But with nothing left to believe in, on what should I base my morality?

'So you're trying to sort out what's right and wrong?'

'Yes. All the time.'

Going to pubs and nightclubs. Smoking. Drinking. Swearing. Petting. I'd rebelled against my religion enough to be doing plenty of those things – but with no real pleasure, just a head full of conflicts and confusion. I felt adrift in a meaningless world.

I stared at an ink stain on his desk. 'Nothing makes sense any more.'

'I see.'

I had difficulty hearing and being heard. Dr Sugden spoke softly, and he'd obviously got a hearing problem. On top of that, I felt intensely shy with him. I could scarcely meet his gaze, and a feeling that I was being prematurely and negatively evaluated added to my discomfort. How much easier it was to talk about these things to Jackie, or even to Pastor West. There was another of many awkward silences, and shyness made me fidget.

'You're not well,' he said. How swiftly a mental illness verdict was reached by a man who had never seen me before in his life. 'You're heading for a nervous breakdown.'

A nervous breakdown? I wasn't sure what that meant but I wondered why I hadn't had one sooner as I'd been like this for such a long time.

'So do I need to stay off work?' I asked. I'd been off work for three weeks, my longest break since starting work at fifteen. I knew I'd better go back soon but I hoped to have just a little more time.

'Yes, and come back to see me next week.'

I walked from the hospital into town where I had tea in a café. Then I went to meet Danny, my latest boyfriend. He had been my favourite singer at the Tempest Folk Club when I was fifteen, but we'd only been dating since we met again about three months before. He'd earned his living by singing in clubs since travelling from his home in Devon, though now he had few bookings and could barely manage to scrape enough money together to live on. But who needs money when you can live on dreams? I thought cynically.

Danny greeted me excitedly. 'I've written another song,' he said, 'and I've got the tune for it worked out on my guitar now. It's dedicated to you. Wanna come to my digs and hear it?'

Listening to Danny singing had never failed to cheer me up before. When he played his guitar and sang, his eyeballs would sometimes disappear up into his forehead leaving only the whites of his eyes showing and, while he was singing lovely romantic songs to me, I'd be trying hard not to laugh. Today, however, I didn't even want to smile when he sang. His cold, shabby bed-sit with its hard, lumpy furniture and peeling damp walls was as bleak as my mood.

We sat cross-legged on the threadbare rug in front of the small gas fire, an old blanket draped around us for much-needed warmth. As we shared a drink of tea in a cracked mug – the only mug he possessed – I wondered how much I could tell him.

'Danny, I've just seen a doctor,' I blurted out, unable to bring myself to say the word 'psychiatrist'. 'He said I'm not well.'

13

'But what's wrong?' he asked, looking concerned.

'Acute depression,' I said, remembering the wording on the medical certificates Dr Russo had given me in the past three weeks.

'What are you depressed about?' He slipped his arm around me and I rested my head on his shoulder.

'It's hard to put into words. I'm just so confused about religion and life and … everything.'

'Things are never as bad as they seem,' he said, stroking my hair. 'I always believe that.'

'Yes, I know *you* do,' I said, wondering when he'd last had a good meal as I glanced round his sparsely furnished room. The shiny guitar looked oddly out of place in the drab surroundings.

At home, later that evening, Mum asked what the psychiatrist had said but, before giving me a chance to reply, added, 'I bet he said you've to go back to work, didn't he?'

'No, he never even mentioned going back to work. He said I'm heading for a nervous breakdown.' I paused for effect. 'I've to see him again next Tuesday. I don't know what'll happen if I have this breakdown thing before then.'

'Don't talk silly,' Mum said. 'There's nowt up with you.'

My last weekend before I 'put my head on the chopping block' (as I later came to see it) was a very 'normal' weekend. No pills taken from Friday night to Monday so that I would feel more like doing things. Saturday morning chatting over coffee with Jackie. Saturday afternoon shopping with Mandy. Saturday night dancing at the Mecca with Danny. Sunday afternoon at the bowling alley with Danny, Mandy and her latest boyfriend Pete. Sunday night dancing at the Mecca again. It only stands out in my memory now because this was to be my last 'ordinary' weekend for a long time.

Although Dad didn't seem to understand why I had decided to see a psychiatrist he was less against the idea than my mother was. On my second visit he said he'd go to the hospital with me and then we could have tea afterwards in our favourite fish and chip café.

Dr Sugden asked me if I still felt the same as I had last week. Of course I still felt the same. I'd been disillusioned and confused about life for the past few years and, not surprisingly, nothing had happened to change that between last Tuesday and this Tuesday. I nodded.

'Right. I think it would be best for you to come into hospital as a voluntary patient,' he said, shuffling some papers on his desk.

'Which hospital?'

'High Royds.'

What? Me? A mental hospital? High Royds was a large, Victorian-built mental hospital on the edge of Ilkley Moor.

'How long for?'

'About a week.'

'What for?'

'A rest and observation.'

I was more surprised than worried by his suggestion. In fact I was hardly worried at all. I welcomed the idea of a break from my family, and thought it might be an interesting experience, if nothing else. Anyway, it was only for about a week, only for a rest and observation. What was there to lose? I was to report to Thornville Ward the next day.

Dr Sugden asked to see my father, who he had noticed was with me this time, while I returned to the waiting area.

Dad took the news badly; there were tears in his eyes when he came out of the consulting room. 'Jean, you won't believe this,' he said in hushed tones, with furtive glances at the other waiting patients. 'He says you're not well. He wants you to go into High Royds.'

'Yeah, I know,' I said. 'I've agreed to it.'

And so I had agreed to put my head on the chopping block. No, I had agreed to spend 'about a week' in a psychiatric hospital for a 'rest and observation'. That was all. No fuss, no drama, no warning bell that I could hear.

Years later I got hold of my case notes and there I could see that Dr Sugden had already decided I was schizophrenic.

Written me up with that label when he first met me.

But I could never have guessed, on that chilly, autumn day, that the system would come down on me like a steamroller; my career as a mental patient was about to take off.

Jackie, who was now off work with her anxiety, called round later that afternoon.

'High Royds? You're joking!' she said.

Even after I managed to convince her it was true, she still seemed to think it was all something of a joke. With an expression of mock seriousness she said, 'Well, yes, Jean, I can just see you basket-making with the loonies.'

We both giggled; it really did seem quite hilarious.

I met Danny that evening and, in the coffee bar at the bowling alley as we waited for a lane, I said, 'Danny, I've got summat to tell you.' I took a deep breath; this wasn't easy. 'I'm going into High Royds tomorrow.'

His mouth dropped open. 'High Royds? Why?'

'The doctor thinks a rest will do me good.'

'A rest? In that place? Why?'

I shrugged my shoulders.

'I ... I don't know what to say,' he said, fiddling with the crucifix on a silver chain he always wore round his neck. 'High Royds? Jesus, that's awful.'

'It's no big deal,' I said. 'It'll only be for about a week.'

'You know what's caused this, don't you?' Mum said tearfully as I packed later that evening. 'It's because of what you did last Thursday night.'

I tried to remember what reckless deed or dreadful sin I'd committed last Thursday night.

'I've told you before. My Great-aunt Annie died when she did that.'

All became clear. I didn't need to ask, 'Did what?' because I remembered the tale of her poor Great-aunt Annie.

'Well, maybe the ceiling fell on her head while she was doing it,' I joked.

'It's nowt to laugh about,' Mum said gravely, but I couldn't stop myself. 'You should never have washed your hair when you was having a period.'

How strange it felt to be packing my clothes into the same suitcase I'd used to go on holiday to Butlins in Skegness with Mandy four months before, when I'd made the decision to visit my GP. The sight of the half-packed case kept playing tricks on my mind, giving me a holiday feeling.

The next day, Wednesday 4 December 1968, I wrote in my diary four little words: 'I'm going in today.'

'I'm warning you,' Mum said, when I was about to set off with Dad, who'd offered to accompany me. 'Once somebody sets foot inside one of those places, they can never get out of their clutches.'

'Oh, Mum, mental hospitals aren't like they were in the olden days,' I said, laughing. 'Some of your ideas come out of the ark.'

'Take no notice of me if you like, but one day you'll remember what I've just said. And you won't be laughing then.'

CASE NO. 10826

Salient Psychiatric Symptoms and Signs on Admission:
Admitted from my clinic at St Luke's Hospital as an informal
patient, where her history clearly indicated that she was
suffering from a schizophrenic type of illness and had been for
some months before. She had been abnormally preoccupied
with questions of a religious character and was morbidly
concerned about questions of right and wrong, to such an
extent that she could not think in a normal way or live a
normal existence. She was markedly introverted with gross
flatenning[sic] of affect. She had obvious difficulty in
concentrating and there was great lack of spontaneity.

Family History:
It seems likely that both the father and the mother are
unstable persons.

Dr Sugden *

* Names of all medical professionals have been changed

CHAPTER TWO

HIGH ROYDS PSYCHIATRIC HOSPITAL, formerly Menston Lunatic Asylum, was situated about seven miles to the north of Bradford, on the edge of Ilkley Moor. Set in spacious grounds, surrounded by sprawling fields, there was once a self-contained community here where inmates could be kept out of sight and mind of the public. I didn't know what to expect as I walked up the long, winding driveway in the fading evening light, my father beside me carrying my case. A sense of foreboding ousted my curiosity as we rounded a bend, for there it stood: large, dark and drear. A Victorian madhouse. I clutched Dad's arm.

On entering, we found ourselves standing on a tiled floor in a stark corridor with high ceiling arches. The air was thick with the smell of cleaning fluid and in the distance I could hear someone crying. A nurse directed us to Thornville Ward.

Thornville was brightly lit, and had potted plants, a radiogram, a TV, tropical fish and a noisy budgie. It was, I understood later, a 'showpiece' ward. I tried not to stare at the occupants of the armchairs seated around the TV, but I was curious to know what these mental patients I had come to stay with were like. They looked like ordinary women, but I thought there must be some strange and terrible sickness lurking behind the façade of normality.

A dumpy nurse with straight black hair introduced herself as Sister Grayston.

'Follow me,' she said, waddling off down the corridor from the day room to the dormitories.

'She looks like a penguin,' my father observed.

'Shh, Dad,' I whispered back, grinning.

She took us to an oblong room, which contained several beds down each side.

'If you've got any valuables you must give them to me for safe keeping,' she explained. Her manner, like her white starched apron, was stiff and practical.

Sister Grayston left my dad and me alone. We sat on the hard bed with its crisp, white sheets and pale-green bedspread. I put the Lucozade my mother had given me on top of the small bedside cabinet next to the Gideon Bible and placed my old, familiar pyjamas, neatly folded, on to my pillow. What was I doing here? My it's-no-big-deal attitude was fast deserting me and I wondered what would happen. But at least it was only for a week, I reminded myself. Only for a week.

'Don't worry, Dad,' I said, squeezing his hand because he looked upset. Focusing on him distracted me briefly from those stabs of anxiety inside me.

After Dad left, Sister Grayston took me to a room at the end of the corridor where I was weighed. I then had to give a urine sample, which wouldn't have been a problem if she hadn't stayed with me. I sat there, bare-arsed, on a commode-like contraption. My body tensed up in embarrassment, adamantly refusing to perform this natural function.

'You said you could do a sample now,' she complained.

'I ... I thought I could,' I said, feeling myself blush.

We both waited in silence, expectantly. Nothing happened.

'Are you going to do anything or not? Hurry up!' she snapped.

I was thankful when she left the room but the sound of her uniform rustling told me she was near and I still couldn't relax sufficiently, even though my bladder felt full to bursting. At last nature took its course, hitting the container noisily and heralding the speedy reappearance of Sister Grayston.

'That's a good girl,' she beamed.

I was sent to join the other patients in the day room, and a small, pasty-faced girl with thick brown hair tied back in a ponytail came and sat next to me. She looked very young.

'It seems strange in here at first,' she said sympathetically. 'I've been in here a few months so I know what's what now. My name's Debbie. I'm thirteen.'

Debbie had the same dull, heavy-lidded eyes as most of the patients, but if she was supposed to be mentally ill I could see no trace of it.

'Have you seen the Quiet Room yet?' she asked.

'The what?'

'The Quiet Room. Come on, I'll show you.'

I followed Debbie down the corridor to a small, carpeted, windowless room containing four brown upholstered chairs with mustard cushions and a low coffee table. The walls were painted that same pale hospital green as the dormitories. On the floor in the corner were a record player and a few pop records.

A tall young woman with blonde curly hair came in. 'Hi, I'm Sheila. Welcome to the nuthouse,' she said, greeting me with a smile. 'I'm glad we've got another young 'un here 'cos most of the others are old fogeys. But perhaps I'm an old fogey to you? I'm twenty-one. I'll guess you're about sixteen.'

'Eighteen,' I said, smiling shyly.

'Pills time again,' Debbie said, standing up at the sound of a rattling, squeaky trolley being wheeled past the door.

Sheila giggled merrily and sang, 'Shake, rattle and roll ...' as she danced down the corridor behind the drugs-laden trolley, but her sad, pale blue eyes belied her show of gaiety.

Before going to bed I was given two large Mogadon sleeping tablets. Despite them, I lay awake for a long time staring up at the dim green ceiling light which stayed on all night. I remembered how way back in childhood we'd talked about men in white coats taking people away in green vans to Menston Loony Bin. So this was Menston. I really was here.

The ward was stirring when I awoke at seven. I followed other sleepy-eyed, dressing-gown-clad patients, clutching plastic toilet bags, down the corridor to a white-tiled room with a row of washbasins. After washing and dressing, I again took my cue from other patients. First there were our beds to make. I pulled the sheets back and, as if I needed a sharp reminder of

21

where I was, there emblazoned in large, black letters across the grey blanket underneath were the words: 'MENSTON HOSPITAL'.

Sister Oldroyd was on duty: a tall, thin woman with heavy black eyeliner drawn around tired eyes. Sitting in the day room before breakfast, a pale, gaunt, elderly patient with sunken grey eyes pointed at my slippers.

'You'll be in trouble if Sister Oldroyd sees you wearing those.'

'Why?'

'You're supposed to wear shoes during the day, luv. That's the rule, and in here you'll keep to the rules without asking questions if you know what's good for you.'

After breakfast Sheila asked me to go to the shop with her. We walked through a maze of long, bleak corridors, which branched off here and there leading to the recesses of the hospital. I was in another world. A world that reeked of cleaning fluid and urine and sadness and pain. A world inhabited by strange men and women who wandered these corridors like the living dead, muttering to themselves, arguing and fighting with their own personal demons, or just staring blankly into space as they shuffled past us with heads down, shoulders drooping: the dejected demeanour of the institutionalised. My heart filled with sadness. How did people end up like that? What had happened to them? Were they once just ordinary babies, children, teenagers? Who were they?

After what must have been the longest indoor walk I'd ever taken, we arrived at the small shop where patients were queuing to buy items such as cigarettes, sweets and tissues. The man behind me in the shop queue stroked my hair, drooling, 'You've got to stroke women, women like to be stroked. Just like this, gently and easily. They like it. You've got to stroke women, women like to be stroked ...'

'Give over,' I said, turning round.

'I'm sorry, young woman, no offence meant,' he mumbled. 'I'm going.'

I watched him shuffling away.

22

We returned to the ward where patients had formed a queue at the trolley to be given drugs. I hung back because Dr Sugden had said I was being admitted for 'a rest and observation'. Nothing had been said about drugs.

'Come on, we haven't got all day,' Sister Oldroyd barked at me. 'What's your name?'

'Jean Davison.'

She fished out an indexed card from a box on the trolley.

'Ah yes, you're on Largactil, seventy-five milligrams three times a day.'

She poured some golden-brown liquid from a large bottle into a small, plastic container. Obediently, I swallowed the medication.

'Where's everybody going?' I asked Debbie who, like the others, was putting on her coat.

'To the therapy block across the grounds,' she replied.

'What's therapy?'

'Don't you know that?' She sounded amazed at such ignorance. 'It's making things. You can learn how to make lampshades, baskets, ashtrays or soft toys.'

The ward emptied of patients except for three old women and me. A nurse sent me to my dormitory where I had to strip to my waist in front of a Dr Prior who placed a stethoscope on my chest and gave me a blood test. Later, I was called to the Quiet Room where he was sitting, feet spread out, smoking a cigarette, and looking at some papers on his knee.

'Sit down,' he said, motioning to the chair facing him. I sat stiffly, perched on the edge of my chair, shyness making me feel ill at ease.

'Relax, I don't bite,' he said, smiling, showing a neat row of gleaming white teeth. He looked to be in his late twenties and wore a grey tweed jacket, crisp white shirt and dark-grey trousers.

'I work under Dr Sugden and I'll be seeing you from time to time. Can you tell me why you're here?'

'Well, for quite some time I've been thinking life seems meaningless and empty.' I stopped. What else was there to say?

Besides, I wasn't in the mood now for talking. I was feeling very sleepy.

He leaned forward in his chair. 'Go on,' he said, nodding encouragingly.

'And I'm confused about religion.'

'Is it very important for you to believe in God?' he asked, looking at the papers on his knee.

'I wish I had summat to believe in.'

'Do you think about religion a lot?'

'Yes.'

'All the time?'

'A lot. Not just about religion. About beliefs generally. I can't sort out what to believe in. I'm confused with so many different ideas.'

'Can you be more specific?'

'I started thinking about lots of things and questioning all me beliefs until I ended up not knowing what to believe in, and it's made me feel kinda lost. I feel as if I don't know what I am.'

He wrote something down, then looked at me. 'When you say you don't know what you are, what exactly do you mean?'

I searched my mind in vain for the words that might get him to understand. 'Oh, I can't explain it any further than that,' I said, feeling weary. 'I don't know how to put these feelings into words.'

'I see,' he said, writing something down. 'So it's as if you've got a thought-block?'

'Is it?' I didn't know if he was asking me or telling me. It was especially difficult for me to find the right words to explain what I meant when trying to talk about personal things to a man I didn't know who was making notes about me. So that was a thought-block? 'Yeah, well I guess I've got plenty of those, then,' I said, managing a smile though I felt embarrassed and nervous.

'You say you don't know what you are. What sort of person do you want to be?'

'I want to be a good Christian,' I said. 'Or at least I thought

I did. But, like I say, I can't believe in the Christian doctrines any more.'

'Is there a particular religious belief that's causing you most problems?'

'Well, it's all of them really, but I can give you an example of one of the teachings which confuses me very much. It's the belief about heaven and hell.'

'Heaven and hell?'

'Yes. It's a belief of the Pentecostal church I used to go to that Christians go to heaven after death and non-Christians go to hell. I can't believe a God of love could send anyone to endless torment.'

He scribbled on his notepad again, then, glancing at his watch, said, 'I must go.' He stood up, flashing a smile. 'I'll see you again soon and we'll have a good talk.'

The other patients came back from therapy at midday. After dinner, the drugs trolley reappeared and we were each given further medication. Visiting time in the afternoon was from two till four. Danny arrived at two. We sat holding hands at a table in the dining area where I struggled to stop my eyelids from slowly closing. I kept glancing at my watch longing for four because I was too drowsy to enjoy a conversation.

'God, they've really doped you, haven't they?'

'Yes, I am very tired. I suppose it must be the drugs.'

A frown crossed his face. He sighed. 'Oh well, they must know what's best for you,' he said.

'Yes, I suppose they do,' I murmured sleepily.

After tea, it was drugs time again, so I swallowed more Largactil syrup, then everyone settled down either to watch TV or to put their heads back in the armchairs and sleep. Evening visiting time was seven till eight. My parents and Danny arrived promptly, but I longed to go to bed and sleep.

When bedtime finally came at nine, I didn't join the queue for sleeping pills until a nurse called me to the trolley.

'Am I supposed to take sleeping pills every night even if I *can* sleep without them?' I ventured to ask her. I could barely manage to keep awake so it seemed absurd.

'Oh yes, it's written on your card,' was her curt reply.

A dark interlude of oblivion. And then morning again. Or something like that. After a drugged sleep, wrenching my head from the pillow was much harder than it had ever been. Groggy and dazed, I pulled on my dressing-gown and stumbled along the corridor to the washroom. There, I let the water from the cold tap run icy cold before splashing it on my face in an attempt to make myself feel somewhere near alive.

After breakfast I joined the queue at the trolley and dutifully swallowed my medication. I stood by the fish tank and watched the fish darting back and forth, round and round, in their glass prison. Utter futility. Then I sank into an armchair and closed my eyes while listening to the budgie beating its wings against the bars and making a lot of noise. It's cruel to put birds in cages, I realised with a jolt. Funny how I'd never thought of that before.

When I opened my eyes the ward had emptied.

'Why aren't you at OT?' a stern voice demanded to know.

'OT?'

'Occupational Therapy,' Sister Grayston informed me. 'Where the other patients are and where you should be too. Off you go.'

The OT building was a place where male and female patients from the various wards came together to engage in activities such as Debbie had described. Miss Burton, the Head Therapist, introduced me to a therapist called Tina, a small, auburn-haired young woman with an old-fashioned beehive hairstyle, who seemed to be attempting something a little more stimulating with a group of about seven teenage patients; it looked like a discussion had been taking place.

Tina pulled a pen and paper from the top pocket of her stiff white overall and added my name to a list.

'This is Jean,' Tina said, addressing the group and motioning me forward. 'Now, Jean, I want you to do some role-play with Peter.'

She placed two chairs in the centre for Peter and me while the rest of the group formed a semi-circle round us.

'What I want you to do, Jean, is to pretend Peter is your fiancé and you've just found out he's a drug addict. OK?'

Peter, a shy-looking, painfully thin, pimply youth of about nineteen looked heavily drugged anyway, which added a touch of reality. He was slouching forward in his chair staring at his shoes. After an awkward silence, I said, 'So you're a drug addict?'

'Yeah,' he replied, without looking up.

'What kind of drugs?'

No reply.

'Well, is it something you swallow or are you injecting?'

Still no reply.

'How long have you been on drugs?'

He shrugged his shoulders.

'Why did you start taking drugs?'

Tina said, 'That's a good question. Now come on, Peter. Tell her why.'

'I ... I don't know,' he said, raising his head just enough for me to see he'd turned crimson. My heart went out to him; he was shyer than I was.

'Do you *want* to come off drugs, Peter?' I asked. 'Are you willing to see a doctor and try to come off them?'

'I don't know,' said Peter. And then we both lapsed into silence. End of act.

Tina clapped her hands.

'That was very good. Tell me, Jean. If he wouldn't come off drugs, would you break off the engagement with him?'

'Yes,' I replied, not giving it much thought. I couldn't imagine being told by someone I knew well and loved that he was a drug addict, and not having had the slightest idea until then.

'Very good,' Tina said again. 'So would I. You'd be well rid of him if he was on drugs.'

Next came a quiz. I was surprised to find that the teenage girl who appeared to be the most severely disturbed patient in

27

our group, Joan, knew more of the answers than any of us. But her answers were interspersed with senseless laughter, tears, screaming, rocking back and forth, asking everyone silly questions and hitting those of us who didn't answer her. This fair-haired, blue-eyed teenager was the disruptive element in the group. The joker was Raymond, aged about eighteen, who kept everyone amused with his own bubbly brand of humour.

'Joan was at grammar school not long ago doing A levels,' Raymond told me at break when we sat together in a corner of the noisy hall sipping stewed tea from badly stained plastic cups. 'She got meningitis. Left her with permanent brain damage.'

'Oh, isn't it sad?'

'Yes, it's sad but that's life,' he said matter-of-factly. 'Anyway, what about you? Can I ask the old corny question: what's a nice girl like you doing in a place like this?'

'Well, I think the diagnosis is acute depression,' I said. 'So perhaps they believe giving me a dose of this dismal place will make me realise I'd got nowt to be sad about before.'

Raymond grinned. He offered me a cigarette.

'No thanks. Tried smoking but gave up while stopping was still easy.'

'Very sensible,' he said, lighting up.

'And you?' I asked. 'Why are you here?'

'Oh, I'm a really bad case.' His dark eyes twinkled. 'I've been here a year.'

'A year!'

'Yeah, well, it's somewhere to live, isn't it? I suppose if I'm a good boy and don't talk as if I might cut my wrists again, I'll eventually return to the big bad world and then ...' His smile faded. 'And then I can do what I want to do with my rotten, lousy, fucked-up life.'

'And what's that?'

'End it.'

'But that wouldn't solve owt, would it?' I put to him hesitantly, aware of the need to tread carefully now that his cheerful mask had slipped.

'It would solve *everything*. But let's quit this morbid talk.' His painted grin returned. 'Do you know any good jokes?'

After tea break I was sent to the therapy workshop where patients were sitting in rows at long workbenches. Here, I was shown how to make an ashtray with small coloured square tiles by tearing off the gauzy backing material which kept the tiles together and then gluing each tile to a metal base. It was dreadfully boring, but there were distractions. Enid, the stout, elderly woman on my right, kept talking to herself. Mary, on my left, shuffled about in her seat, sometimes clapping her hands while she laughed and laughed.

Occasionally I glanced at Fred opposite to see if he still kept breaking off from the basket he was making to pull faces or wink at me. Only a few days ago I'd been laughing with Jackie when we'd joked about me sitting 'basket-making with the loonies'. It didn't seem funny now. Nothing seemed funny now.

CASE NO. 10826

Mental state:
Young apprehensive girl, reasonably well dressed and co-operative and pleasant.
Capable of holding good stream of conversation. Finds it difficult to express herself of the thought disorder – as she cannot express the feelings in words.

Thought disorder of bizarre in[sic] nature:
'I am confused with so many different ideas.' 'Heaven and hell confuses me very much.' 'I do not know <u>what</u> I am at times,' etc. Expresses these thoughts with particular reference to religion – 'I want to be a good Christian.'

Perceptual disturbance:
Absent.

Passivity feeling perhaps present:
Not deluded with depersonalisation.
Orientation: full. Memory – Intact.

General Informations:
Intact.

Schizophrenia (Simplex) in a young girl with ? family history.

Dr Prior

CHAPTER THREE

THE FIRST FEW DAYS in High Royds passed in a blur. My thoughts became fuzzy as the drugs took a firm hold, and I sank into the regimented routine of the institution. Up at seven. Bed at nine. And in between, a drowsy dream-state of longing for bedtime. I would wake in the morning to face another day stretching ahead of me like an endless, gloomy tunnel.

At OT, I sometimes escaped from the monotony of knitting dishcloths and making ashtrays by lingering in the toilet. The door wouldn't lock but a measure of privacy for writing could be achieved by sitting on the floor with knees to chest, feet against the base of the pot and back against the door holding it firmly shut. This was where I sat, scribbling copious notes for my diary, pouring my heart out on wads of toilet paper.

I was standing alone among the crowd of patients in the therapy hall at tea break watching a tall, wiry woman with a 'basin' haircut on what seemed to be her daily scrounge for cigarettes.

'Have you got a cig?' she asked.

I shook my head. 'I don't smoke.'

She eyed me up and down whilst nervously twisting a lock of hair around her shaky, nicotine-stained fingers, with nails bitten to the quick.

'I'm Beryl. What's your name?'

'Jean.'

'How old are you?'

'Eighteen.'

'Oh dear, oh dear, I thought so. I knew it,' she said,

frowning. 'I can see it all again now.'

The way she was staring at me and shaking her head mournfully made me feel uncomfortable.

'You remind me of myself about thirty years ago. This is your first time in a mental hospital, isn't it?'

I nodded.

'Yes, like me. I was eighteen. I've been in and out ever since and I expect I'll be a permanent resident now. It all starts when you first come in. Once you're in, they've got you.'

This reminded me of my mother's warning that you'd never get away once they got their clutches on you. But what did my mother know about it? As for Beryl, well, surely this was her illness talking, and of course it was completely different for me.

Beryl's eyes darted back and forth like a trapped animal. 'It's like being in prison, only worse. You'll see.'

'I'm a voluntary patient,' I informed her.

'Voluntary. Ah, yes,' she said with a strange, crooked smile. 'What does that word mean in here?' Her breath was coming out in noisy puffs; she seemed very agitated. 'Have they given you any treatment yet?'

'Just drugs.'

'Yes, like me. First the pills. Lots of pills. Make you very sleepy, don't they? Have they given you electric shock treatment yet?'

'Electric shock treatment?'

'Yes. They zap your brain with electric.' She pointed a finger to her head like a gun. 'Pow! It's supposed to shock you back into sanity by destroying your brain cells.'

'No, I'm not having that. I only came in for about a week, so I'll be going home in a couple of days.'

'Oh, sure you will. Is that what they told you? They told me that, too. I was only eighteen. You're only eighteen. It's terribly sad. I hope you'll be OK but I know how it can happen and …' She bent her face near to my mine. 'I'm scared for you, Jean. Really scared for you.'

My God, what a Job's comforter, I thought as I watched her

shuffling away, stopping every now and then to rummage through ashtrays for tab ends.

When Dr Prior asked to see me in the Quiet Room I thought it must be for the 'good talk' he'd promised, but he said, 'I'll only keep you a moment. First, how are you?'

'Will you cut down me drugs?' I begged him. 'They're making me too drowsy.'

'Drowsiness is not a serious side effect,' he said, lighting a cigarette.

'But it's *awful* being so tired,' I pointed out, exasperated.

'Well, just lie on your bed for a while when you feel tired.'

How I wished I could. He obviously wasn't aware of the rules.

'Do you enjoy going to OT?' he asked, changing the subject.

'I'm so tired and bored there. Do I *have* to go?'

'No, not if you don't want to.'

'Oh, thank you,' I said, grateful for small mercies. Sitting in rows at the therapy workbenches reminded me of the factory assembly line, except it was even worse. In the factory each minute had passed, albeit slowly, but at OT it was as if time just hung about sleepily and lingered in the air mingling with the atmosphere of deep gloom that clung to the walls and ceiling, enfolded us like a shroud and dampened at source any spark of humour. It was the same in the ward to some extent, but nowhere had I experienced it more keenly than in the OT department.

'Now, listen to me, Jean,' Dr Prior was saying. 'I'd like you to have a course of about six to eight applications of electric shock treatment. Don't let the term "electric shock" frighten you. It's a safe, simple procedure. A small electric current is passed through your brain but it's all done under anaesthetic so you won't feel a thing.'

It was a bit better than Beryl's version, but I still didn't like the sound of it.

'We don't know how it works,' he said. 'Only that

somehow it shakes the mind up, lifting depression and enabling a patient to think clearly.'

But I needed to think clearly now, so that I could understand what he was suggesting. And thinking clearly was far from easy when I was heavily drugged.

'I can't see how it could help me,' I said, feeling puzzled.

'Well, I think we should at least give it a try. Now if you'll just sign this, please.'

He produced a printed form from his briefcase and handed it to me with a pen. I read: 'As this form of treatment is not without an element of risk we should like to have your consent to employ it ...'

As I tried to decide what to do, Dr Prior waved his hand. 'This paper's just a formality: there's really no need to read it.'

'What's the risk?' I asked, as this was not explained on the form.

'There is no risk,' he replied.

I felt decidedly uneasy. He was telling me that the form did not mean what it said, was unimportant, and that it was unnecessary for me even to read it – but nonetheless my signature was required on it. I began reading it again while trying to ignore Dr Prior who kept impatiently pointing to the space at the bottom where he wanted me to sign. *As this form of treatment is not without an element of risk ...*

'Why does it say there is a risk if there isn't?' I persisted.

'It says what? Let me see that form.' He looked at it and frowned. 'Oh, damn! I've given you the wrong one,' he said. 'Not to worry though. I'll just amend it slightly then you can sign it.'

He made some minor adjustments, as the form had obviously been designed for someone to sign on behalf of the patient, then he handed it back to me.

'What's the risk?' I asked again. 'It says there is an element of risk.'

He drew heavily on his cigarette, and sighed. 'The risk is in the anaesthetic, not the treatment,' he said, 'and all anaesthetics carry an element of risk but it's so slight that it's not worth worrying about. You don't worry each time you cross a road but there's far more risk in that. Now, just sign it there.'

I studied his face carefully, wondering why he seemed impatient and evasive. I looked back down at the form. The words were blurred; my eyesight, previously excellent, had deteriorated rapidly in the few days since my admission, presumably due to the drugs. And I was so, so tired. In this strange mental hospital world, one's self-determination and resistance could easily become dangerously low.

'I only want to help you,' Dr Prior was saying. 'You do trust me, Jean, don't you?'

I still didn't understand. But surely I could trust professional medical staff who wanted to help me.

'Yes, I trust you,' I said weakly, as he pushed the pen into my hand.

I no longer trusted God. I no longer trusted my own thoughts and feelings. I supposed I had to trust somebody. So I signed.

'That's a good girl,' Dr Prior said, smiling.

Good girl? Naughty girl? It didn't matter whether a patient was thirteen or seventy-plus or anything in between, psychiatric staff still persisted in talking to us in those terms.

Many years later I saw again the consent form I'd signed and remembered how Dr Prior, before realising he'd given me the wrong form, had said emphatically: 'There is no risk.' There was also a form signed by another patient that day which had obviously been filed into my case notes by mistake. On this, there was no mention of 'risk'. Instead, it emphasised that an assurance had 'NOT' been given that the treatment would be administered by a specific practitioner (surely ironically irrelevant to most patients in the circumstances).

Instead of setting off for OT the next day, I remained in the day room and started writing a letter to Mandy.

'What do you think you're doing?' You should be at OT,' Sister Oldroyd snapped at me.

'Dr Prior says I don't have to go to OT,' I said innocently.

I could never have guessed the effect of these words. She actually shook with anger and her voice rose to a shriek as she informed me it made no difference what Dr Prior had said: it was none of his business! It was what Dr Sugden said that counted and he would listen to her about what she thought was good for me, and how dare I sit there and be cheeky enough to say I didn't have to go? If I didn't get out of her sight this minute and off to the OT block, she wouldn't be held responsible for what she'd do to me. Who did the little madam think she was to expect special treatment compared to other patients?

I stood up immediately to fetch my coat. And off the little madam went to OT.

I woke up early the next morning despite the drugs and, fixing my eyes on the green light above, I thought: Today they are going to shoot electric currents into my brain. Why?

I had to get up at seven but remain in my dressing-gown and have nothing to eat or drink. The next three hours were spent sitting in the day room silently waiting, and wishing the sky would fall to stop the day.

The ambulance to take me to the ECT Unit arrived at ten. Inside were six women from other wards wearing dressing-gowns, and two young nurses. As we rode across the broken tarmac in the grounds the two nurses joked with each other while we, the victims of God knew what, sat silently, squashed together, alone with our 'sick' thoughts.

We jerked to a stop outside a heavy wooden door and were ushered into the building. One sharp breath of fresh, winter air and then a stuffy warmth again with a faint smell of the now familiar cleaning fluid. I tried to understand this 'sickness' of mine. Was I a troubled teenager or a hard-core psychotic? In this mental hospital there was, apparently, no distinction. We were heavily drugged, categorised as 'sick', sat side by side making ashtrays and knitting dishcloths. Perhaps, too, we were all experiencing the same naked fear as we sat together on the wooden bench in this small, oblong waiting area.

The elderly and most confused patients were frisked to check that all hairgrips, false teeth, glasses and anything with metal fasteners had been removed. A nurse appeared with a syringe to give us an injection in the arm; a procedure which proved difficult since some of the patients chose to engage her in a cat-and-mouse game. I was one of the good, co-operative patients who smiled for the benefit of some frightened patients who were studying my face as she pushed the needle in.

'What's the injection for?' someone asked.

'It's to dry your mouth so you don't swallow your tongue and choke to death while you're having a fit,' the nurse explained coolly. 'So if you don't let me give you it you might die.'

'Do you think that bothers us, you fool? We all want to die.'

I tried to say, 'No, not all of us. I don't want to die,' but the words froze on my lips and I couldn't speak.

After the injection came a half-hour anxiety-filled period of waiting, during which time there was nothing to do but sit and think. I thought about how my hospital stay was meant to be for a week. In my sleepy state it was hard to keep pace with what was happening to me. Without protest, or even much thought about it, I had resigned myself to a longer stay.

And then my thoughts travelled back to what I was doing a thousand years ago. No, wait a minute; it wasn't really long ago. Today was Thursday and a week last Saturday I was dancing at the Mecca with Danny, then on the Sunday afternoon Danny and I went to the bowling alley with Mandy and Pete and, on the Sunday night, we were dancing at the Mecca again. Then on the Tuesday, the evening before my admission, I was at the bowling alley with Danny. So that must have been … I counted the days backwards on my fingers … Nine days ago! How could that be? Only nine days ago. Another place. Another world.

As the time for 'treatment' drew near we took turns to go to the toilets in the wooden cubicles with three-quarter-length doors that wouldn't lock, and then a nurse passed a hot-water bottle round which was placed on the back of our hand to try to get the vein to stand out clearly. By this time my tongue felt too big to fit properly inside my dry mouth, my throat was parched, and I could hardly swallow.

Another nurse appeared with a sheet of paper. She gave us each a number, arranging us to sit in a certain order. I was Number Seven. I used to think seven was a lucky number when I was a little girl. I remembered how it had once won me a huge box of chocolates tied with a red ribbon in a raffle. Strange how often irrelevant thoughts intrude at moments of crisis in our lives. All Number Seven meant to me now was that my agony of waiting was to be prolonged because I was the last in the queue.

The nurse escorted Number One away. They disappeared through a double door. Silence fell over the waiting group, then someone said: 'Oh God, we're lined up like sheep for the slaughter!'

My heart was thudding wildly as I stared at the closed door. It was about to begin.

A few minutes after the nurse and Number One left, a scream like something out of a horror film resounded from the adjoining treatment room.

'I'm going home,' announced a middle-aged woman, standing up. She was Number Two.

'Home? Like that, in your dressing-gown and slippers? You won't get far, luv,' smiled the male attendant who had been assigned to watch over us. It was Number Two's turn next but she had run off down the corridor and was trying frantically to open the outer door to go 'home'. The attendant brought her back. 'Sit down luv. You *are* home.'

Number Two sat down in her allocated position, placid now, saying, 'This is my home? Oh Lord in heaven, help us all.'

One by one we were led through the door from where the screams came. Never before had I felt more vulnerable than I did lying on my back, with a white-coated man bending over me, ready to interfere with my brain. I must be far sicker than I realised, so I've just got to trust them, I thought achingly, through the Largactil haze.

'Count to ten,' the white-coated man said as he pricked the vein in the back of my hand, which stood up prominently after the heat of the hot-water bottle. One. Two. Three. Four ... A strange, onion-like smell clogged my nostrils and filled my head, sending my senses reeling violently. Up till then I'd been lying co-operatively and still, but now this dreadful sensation brought on a surge of panic and I struggled like a demon.

'Naughty, naughty girl,' a distant voice was saying – just like the school dentist had said when I'd fought him while being given gas. Don't let them do this to you, don't let them do it, a part of my mind was screaming. I was rigid with terror, knowing I *must* stop them. I *must*. I *must* ... But someone or something was holding me down firmly in a suffocating blackness as dark as the grave. I couldn't move, couldn't see, couldn't breathe. Powerless, overcome, I was hurled into oblivion.

CHAPTER FOUR

IT WAS NEARLY CHRISTMAS and I wanted nothing to do with it. Brightly coloured paper trimmings, streamers and balloons were festooned on the walls and ceiling, looking as false to me as the false hope they symbolised. If we need an excuse for eating too much or getting drunk, then why not call it celebrating the birth of a long dead Saviour, I thought cynically as I gazed at the large Christmas tree in the hall at OT with its silly baubles and stupid star on top; this farce called Christmas left me cold. But when we made trimmings – coloured paper chains from strips of gummed paper just as I'd done as a child – I wanted to cry: it was the happy, not sad, memories of the past which now pained me most of all.

One afternoon at OT we were herded into the main hall to sing carols. At break Joan stood in front of me. 'If they had known Jesus was the Son of God, they wouldn't have crucified him, would they?' Her fists were clenched ready to thump me if I didn't answer.

'I don't know.'

'But they wouldn't, would they?'

She was making me think, damn her. I was too tired to think.

'I don't know, Joan.'

She raised her fists higher. 'Yes, you *do* know,' she shrieked. 'They wouldn't. Would they?'

'No, Joan, I don't suppose they would.'

'Then why didn't they know He was the Son of God?'

And so it went on.

After break we resumed singing. Joan, who was sitting next

to me now, was laughing and muttering senselessly as one possessed. My mind travelled back to two Christmases ago when I had sung these same carols in the bright, cheery atmosphere of the church Youth Leader's house. I hadn't thought then that I would end up in here. But I hadn't thought a lot of things then.

I had leave from the hospital for a few days at Christmas. My parents were given little plastic containers of pills to last me until my return on Boxing Day.

At home my brother the bus conductor sneered. 'People think you're a nutcase when I tell them you're in High Royds. The bus drivers and conductors on this route all know, 'cos why should I keep it secret?'

'You can shout it through a loudspeaker from the rooftop for all I care,' I said wearily, 'but they'll think it's you who's the nutcase for wanting to tell everyone.'

'It's not just you he talks about,' put in my father. 'He tells people when me and your mum haven't slept together. Everyone knows our business, whenever we row, everything. People do think there's summat wrong with Brian, and I think so too.'

'Well, *I'm* the one who's in High Royds.' I was aware that a note of bitterness had crept into my voice.

'I can't understand why,' Dad said. 'You're the sanest person in this family. Brian's certainly got no sense.'

'I've got more sense than Jean. *I'm* not a mental patient. Tell me, Jean, how does it feel to be a mental case?' He grinned fiendishly then began tapping with a spoon on a milk bottle, but stopped when Dad threatened to knock his head off his shoulders.

I went upstairs and transferred what I'd written on scraps of toilet roll at the hospital into my diary. I'd kept a diary for many years. Writing things down helped me to sort out my thoughts and feelings. It seemed important to try to continue doing this.

I spent Christmas in bed sleeping, or sitting around the

house in my dressing-gown, face unwashed, hair unkempt. I was aware that my life was drifting downhill, but lacked the energy or motivation to exert myself. In this state I just took it for granted that I would return to the hospital after the holiday. My parents also accepted this, as was their way. There was one bright spot. Jackie called to see me. She had stopped taking her tranquillisers and looked well and happy. I was worlds of experience away from the teenager I'd been when I'd last seen her before my admission only three weeks ago, so it was encouraging to find I could still relate easily to her. My old sense of humour even peeped out of its hiding place. Perhaps things weren't really so bad, I began to think hopefully. But the hope was stillborn.

Back in hospital after Christmas, far from my drugs being decreased as I'd hoped, they were intensified, and I felt like a zombie. Truly, I had never felt worse, never even realised before that it was possible to feel so low.

My parents visited and I could barely keep awake when trying to talk with them. I asked them to tell my psychiatrist that the drugs were too strong for me and he needed to decrease them.

'But what can we do now you're in here?' Mum said. Her face looked pale and strained.

I turned to Dad, but he shook his head. 'Jean, love, he's the doctor. We can't tell him what to do.'

Apparently my parents hadn't even thought of asking to speak to my doctor. Danny had told them he felt they should do, and I think they were genuinely puzzled at Danny's insistence. This was the sixties and my parents' attitude towards the medical profession was probably no different from many working-class parents of that time.

A few days later Dr Prior saw me in the Quiet Room for a consultation.

'*Please* will you lower my drugs?' I pleaded with him.

'Not yet,' he said.

'I can't stand it!' I said, a note of despair creeping into my voice.

'What can't you stand?'

'The way the drugs make me feel. Being in this place. I can't mix with people so I feel isolated.'

'Why can't you mix with people?'

'Shyness. And I'm so drowsy I can't think straight.'

'Are you still confused about religion?'

'Yes.' What did he expect me to say? I'd probably be confused about religion for the rest of my life.

'Do you still feel as if you don't know who or what you are?'

'Yes, I do,' I admitted, though I wished I'd never mentioned this or religion in the first place. He wrote something down.

'Will you reduce my tablets?' I begged again. Having to endure this drug-induced lethargy while not being allowed to lie on my bed and sleep all the time was too much to bear. I was desperate. But he just sat there, cold and unmoveable, as he observed my distress.

'Can I be discharged?' I was a voluntary patient but I felt like a prisoner. Living with my family was no real freedom either but it had to be better than this. Yet so subdued was I that I seemed to have acquired a prisoner mentality: it didn't even occur to me to attempt to leave the hospital without permission.

'You're not ready to be discharged.'

'But I can't stand it!' I said again, unable to contain my anguish.

He added something to his notes, replaced the cap on his pen and stood up. 'I'll see you again soon,' he said.

Staying awake while doped up with drugs was like an endurance test and my reward for getting through the day was being allowed to go to bed. Sometimes, curled up in bed, I would stare at the green light above and wish I could stay awake long enough to try to understand what was happening to me. But the drugs deadened my brain. I would fall asleep almost immediately unless there was some kind of night-time distraction, such as, for instance, the night Connie left her bed next to mine to climb in with me, subjecting me to sexual advances. She was heavy, physically stronger than me and I was too tired to fight. She lay on top of me, fondling my breasts and kissing my lips while I, loathing every moment, waited for her to shift.

In the morning when making my bed I couldn't remember how to do the corners of the bedspread, which had to be folded a certain way. Sister Grayston came and stood beside me with hands on her hips, watching my fumbling attempt.

'Oh, for goodness' sake!' she said. 'I've already shown you.'

I watched closely while she showed me again, but I felt so heavy and slow that even learning this simple task was difficult. Dr Prior had promised the shock treatment wouldn't impair my intelligence but I knew something was having a detrimental effect.

It had been decided that I would spend most of my OT time in the 'office skills' class to practise typing and learn shorthand. I usually missed this on ECT mornings but once, when I arrived back at the ward after ECT a bit earlier than usual, Sister Oldroyd sent me to the OT department. ECT might cast out conscious knowledge of *some* experiences, whether good or bad, driving them into a deep, secret place beyond recall. But never, never, will I forget the horror and dismay of staring at a page of shorthand symbols that day with the realisation that my ability to think clearly and retain information had been severely, and I feared permanently, impaired.

I kept forgetting how to make those 'hospital corners' with the bedspread, so the routine became that each morning when Sister Grayston was on duty she would stand at the door of my dormitory watching me try. This made me nervous, increasing the likelihood of my getting it wrong.

'Don't you know how to make a bed?' her voice would boom across the room, grating its way into my groggy head.

'How old are you?'

She knew my age, of course, but always pressed me to tell her at this point, then she would tut and say: 'What? Did I hear you right? Eighteen years old and you can't even make a bed?'

I think after a while it must have really got to me; I remember answering 'Eighteen' in a barely audible voice, feeling full of embarrassment and shame at what a stupid girl I must be.

Sister Grayston was a strict, school-marm type, and I didn't like her for humiliating me over the bedspread corners, but I still preferred it when she was on duty rather than Sister Oldroyd.

Sister Oldroyd stopped me one morning while I was walking past her office on my way to the bathroom.

'I'm sick and tired of your attitude,' she snapped. 'You must be in need of help or you wouldn't be here.'

'I am in need of help,' I agreed, feeling bewildered.

'There you are. You're in need of help. You've just said so yourself now. You've admitted it.' She said this gloating in the way of people who feel their opponents in a debate have just tripped themselves up and ruined their own argument. It made no sense to me. I'd sought help myself and agreed to be admitted against the wishes of my parents. Since my admission, I had co-operated with whatever treatment had been prescribed. Not once had I denied I was in need of help.

'I've never said I don't need help,' I said.

'Well, if you admit it, then why have you got that attitude?'

'What attitude?'

'Thinking you're better than everyone else, for one thing.'

This hurt. Penny, a girl at school and Joanne at the television factory, and no doubt countless others, had mistaken my shyness for something else.

'I've never thought that.'

'You've been aggressive since you came here. You've got a chip on your shoulder. Your trouble is that you think everyone is against you.'

Abruptly, she turned and walked away.

45

I was attacked by a patient at OT. Rosie flew at me, shrieking and scratching like a wild cat. She yelled that I'd been staring at her, but I hadn't even noticed her until then. The rest of the noise died down at once and only Rosie's screams of fury could be heard. She was a tall, stout woman but apparently not very strong and, by grasping then holding firmly both her wrists, I was able to restrain her until two white-coated male attendants, who suddenly seemed to appear from nowhere, led her away.

The Head Therapist, Mrs Burton, sat down beside me. 'I'm terribly sorry about this,' she said. 'We know it wasn't your fault. Rosie thinks people are against her. She can't help it because she's very sick. This incident will be reported and Rosie will be punished.'

I wondered why Rosie should be punished for being 'sick'.

I was called from OT because my 'vicar' was waiting to see me. When I arrived back on the ward, Pastor West had been shown into the Quiet Room. I paused with my hand on the doorknob, suddenly feeling nervous. How much had I changed since he'd seen me at home before my admission only a few weeks ago? Did I *look* like a mental patient now? Or was the change only on the inside?

Then a strange thing happened to me. I began shaking all over, as if a pneumatic drill was at work inside me. Feeling embarrassed, I sat in the chair opposite him while he looked surprised and concerned.

'How long have you been like this?'

'It's just started now,' I said, panic rising in me as I tried in vain to regain control over my shaking body. 'It's because you're here.'

'Why do you think that?' he asked, his eyebrows arching into a puzzled frown.

'Because my mind associates you with church, and church with conflict,' I replied unhesitatingly, convinced this was the reason.

'Yes, perhaps so,' Pastor West said slowly. He looked

thoughtful for a moment. 'But you weren't like this when I saw you recently at home, were you?'

He was right. I searched my mind for another explanation. Was it a subconscious way of trying to say to him: 'Look at me. See how desperately I need help now. Why won't your God help me?' Or was it the drugs?

'Well, perhaps it's a side effect of the drugs that's just started up,' I said.

Although not usually so visible, the shakiness was to continue. I came to see it as a symptom of illness but learnt, much later, it was caused by neuroleptic medication.

'Have they put *you* on drugs?' he asked.

'Of course,' I replied, wondering at his surprise. Everyone in my ward was on drugs and I'd already forgotten how I'd been surprised when first given them.

'I'm also having electric shock treatment,' I announced flatly, staring at the floor.

'Shock treatment? But, why?'

'I'm in need of help.'

This conversation was strained, difficult, unlike all our previous chats when I'd entered into lively discussion. I must have looked a total wreck shaking like that and I was aware that I was nervously twisting my long, greasy hair around my trembling fingers as Beryl had done. But what did it matter if I was looking and behaving like a mental patient? I was one.

'I'm going insane,' I said, bending forward and covering my face with my hands.

'Nonsense!' Pastor West said. 'You're as sane as I am.' He paused, then added, 'Though, heaven knows, I don't know if that's any consolation to you.' This made me smile in spite of myself.

'I'm in need of help,' I said again.

'Jean, why do you keep saying you're in need of help?'

'Have I ever seemed aggressive?' I asked.

'Aggressive? Definitely not,' he replied. 'It's not in your nature to be aggressive.'

'Well, have I ever given you the impression that I've a chip on my shoulder or that I feel everyone is against me?'

'No, not at all,' he said. 'Why are you asking?'

I was asking because I was trying to understand Sister Oldroyd's comments. I was asking because I couldn't see why I was being given ECT and drugs. I was asking because I was trying to salvage something of my crumbling sense of identity.

'Oh, it doesn't matter,' I said. 'It's not important.'

After tea I saw the three patients nearest to my age, Maria, Sheila and Tessa, go into the Quiet Room. Knowing what I must do, I didn't allow myself to pause at the door, lest my courage would fail me.

'Mind if I join you?' I asked, trying to sound casual, as three pairs of eyes looked at me. They greeted me with friendly smiles and didn't seem to notice how awkward and shy I was feeling. I began to relax. We were sitting on the floor looking through some pop records discussing our favourites when Connie stuck her head round the door and said Sister Oldroyd was looking for me. Sheila grinned when I pulled a face. 'She's a right cow, isn't she? We've noticed how she picks on you.'

'If she picked on me like that I'd tell her to bleedin' piss off,' said Maria, the girl who, a few days earlier, had been proclaiming she'd had intercourse with God at Lourdes and was the chosen vessel for the second birth of Jesus.

Sister Oldroyd opened the door and glared at me. 'So there you are. Go get a bath. It's been filled.'

Most of the other patients, it seemed, simply told a nurse when they wanted a bath and I, too, would have bathed regularly without needing to be told, but she always sought me out like this. Today it was particularly annoying because I so much wanted to stay and talk with the others, having at last found the courage to approach them. But I sighed and obeyed. After all, what point was there in arguing? What point was there in anything?

When I'd been packing my case to come into hospital I'd packed my favourite soap, talc and perfumed bubble bath. How ridiculously unnecessary these things seemed now, for having a bath was no longer the leisurely, lingering pleasure I'd previously enjoyed. The first time I'd entered the bathroom I'd been disconcerted to find I couldn't lock the door, nor could I get any water out of the bath taps to adjust the temperature of the already filled bath. No sooner had I stripped naked when a confused patient wandered in and out of the bathroom. Then Sister Oldroyd peered round the door and stood there for a while, silently staring at me as I eased myself into the water. Shortly afterwards, a nurse came with scissors and asked if my toenails needed cutting. I hated these humiliating, and in my case needless, invasions of privacy. Privacy: perhaps I shouldn't have expected anything so precious as that in a mental hospital.

One day Lynette, a small hunch-backed woman sitting opposite me, refused to eat her dinner, saying she felt unwell. Sister Oldroyd tried to ram food down her throat then, to my surprise and horror, when Lynette vomited into the food on her plate, attempted to force-feed this back to her before dragging her, screaming and crying, from the dining area.

I stared down at my plate eating mechanically, desperately trying to ignore the stench of vomit wafting up my nostrils, so fearful was I of feeling unable to eat and being dealt with in the same way. Along with nausea and anger I felt a sense of shame to discover that I was capable of witnessing such assaults on another person without taking action. Should I have intervened? But how could I?

I was leaving the medication trolley after taking my pills when Sister Oldroyd swooped on me and opened my hand, almost clawing insanely at my palm, in an attempt to snatch something from it that was not there. On finding nothing, she looked surprised, hesitated, then grabbed and opened my other hand. After eyeing me up and down suspiciously, she abruptly turned and walked away. I was aware of the other patients looking at me and felt hot with embarrassment at becoming the centre of attention.

Sister Oldroyd's job was obviously having an adverse effect

on her. Of course we were all bound to have an effect on each other – staff on patients, patients on staff, patients on patients. But at least the staff could go home when their shift was over, whereas patients remained in close proximity at all times.

An argument between two patients progressed one teatime from shouting across the tables to throwing crockery. Lynette started crying but Andrea smiled complacently as a flying saucer whizzed past her ear. She told us, almost proudly I thought, that this was nothing compared to the fights in a ward where she was once transferred after trying to hang herself with a scarf.

It was surprising that there weren't more fights even in our showpiece ward, considering the stress we were under, herded together day after day in such an unnatural environment. Perhaps the humiliation of being under the supreme power of the staff kept us all subdued and passive.

Remains rather withdrawn; not so preoccupied with religious conflicts. Thought problems are not very prominent but still disturbs the patient – 'I do not yet know – who am I', 'Confused about heaven and hell' etc. Seemed to be more concerned about not being able to mix well. Prominent thought-block is being expressed with distress. Has gained some insight but not sufficiently. Asking for discharge. She is taking very little interest at the occupational therapy or the ward routine.

Dr Prior

CHAPTER FIVE

TWICE A WEEK I received electrical assaults on my brain. Lightning flashes. Convulsions. Blast it all out, forget everything. I slipped off the ladder and couldn't stop falling. I awoke the same but not the same. A searing pain inside my brain. Branded.

I heard someone moaning when they were being given ECT. I was sitting outside the treatment room, nervously twisting my fingers and thinking of the Simon and Garfunkel song 'I Am a Rock' as I awaited my turn.

'Don't worry,' a nurse said to me. 'She can't feel a thing because she's unconscious.'

The moans were terrible; the most poignant, eerie sounds of protest I'd ever heard, springing deep from a woman's unconscious mind. Would I soon be moaning like that? Even the rocks can't remain silent.

During one ECT session there was a group of students peering over me ready to watch my convulsions. Just before being seized by the dreadfully unpleasant sensation I always experienced in the seconds before losing consciousness, a wave of resentment hit me as I gazed up at the sea of curious faces. But I resisted the temptation to yell at them: 'I hope you enjoy the goddamn show!'

It was at the ECT block where I saw thirteen-year-old Debbie again, who had been moved to another ward. At first I didn't recognise the pathetic, drooping figure who was sitting in the waiting area, white-faced and trembling.

'Now don't be silly, dearie,' a stiff-uniformed nurse was saying, offering a tissue to Debbie. 'It's nothing to be scared of. You won't feel a thing.'

'It's all right for *you* to say that,' a small, shaky voice protested. 'You've never had ECT, have you?'

'No, but I do know what I'm talking about,' the nurse said, confident in her textbook knowledge. How could she know, damn her? I thought indignantly. How *could* she know?

My heart cried out with pity for Debbie who knew so much so soon. What, in the name of sanity, was she doing in this place? Dear God, she was only a child.

My fear of ECT gave birth to a gut-twisting anxiety. Admittedly, the treatment itself, being administered when anaesthetised, was painless. But imprinted in my memory is the sensation of lying helplessly as the injected anaesthetic seared my brain and played havoc with my senses before the blackness of oblivion. I tried hard to remain relaxed after being given the anaesthetic but that was like trying to suppress a strong survival instinct; not once did I succeed in 'going gently' into the night.

Next come the after-effects; the post-ECT fog. It's bad enough being given drugs every day, which make you feel dim-witted and slow, but add to this the disorientation following an ECT session and you're living through a nightmare. First, you wake up and wander round with other confused, dressing-gown-clad patients in a daze, not knowing what day it is, what time it is or where the hell you are in this planet of pain. You try to think clearly, realise you can't and fear you must have finally gone completely crazy. Back in the ward, it's difficult to remember the simplest of things, such as the location of your locker, bed or the toilet. You don't want dinner. If you can manage it while Sister isn't looking, and if you can remember where it is, you empty your food into the slop bin, but then the after-dinner drugs rumble around queasily in your empty stomach. Along with your usual drugs there are two extra pills. These are painkillers, which are supposed to take away that dull, sickening pain inside your head, but you're lucky if they touch it. You long to lie on your bed, to escape in sleep, but instead you must face your usual afternoon stint at OT.

And sometimes, while still in this post-ECT fuddle, you wonder what they are doing to your brain. Poor brain. Doped and shocked. Numbed and stunned. Has it been damaged? The mental hospital environment is one that can greatly endanger a person's physical and psychological well-being; that's not being paranoid, it is a fact.

'What can I do? They are trying to kill me,' says Eric, a young man I see at OT who, I think, has been given a 'paranoid schizophrenic' label. 'They watch me closely to make sure I swallow the poison and if that doesn't work then they'll do it by electrocution. If I don't kill myself, they'll murder me.'

Eric must be very sick to talk like that, I realise, and yet his words do seem to make sense in this place. More sense than the words of the staff. I sympathise with Eric's dilemma.

Meanwhile, Mabel rocks back and forth, Deirdre mutters obscenities, Mary laughs and laughs, Lilly sucks her thumb for comfort and Gary plays with his genitals. I am sitting quietly staring down at the small coloured tiles on the workbench used for making ashtrays or sticking on to bottles to make table-lamp stands. I am remembering how, when first admitted, I looked for signs of sickness in other patients behind what I thought was a façade of normality, but now I find it easier, even when watching patients displaying bizarre behaviour, to see the 'normality' behind the 'sickness'. Normality? Sickness? What do these words mean? As I stare at the tiles till their colours blur together, I am coming to believe that the dividing line between 'normality' and 'mental illness' is a very fine one.

Danny came to visit me one afternoon when, only a few hours earlier, I'd been given ECT. I tried to pull my thoughts together to make sensible conversation with him.

'Yes, I know. You've already told me that a few minutes ago,' he said, his soft brown eyes full of pity.

'It's the ECT,' I explained quickly, anxious to let him know I wasn't crazy. 'It makes you forget things, but only temporarily.' At least I hoped the way I felt would be only temporary.

I remembered how before my admission Dr Sugden had said I was 'heading for' a nervous breakdown. That's why he'd wanted me to come into hospital, wasn't it?

'Danny, I'm scared that I'll go ... that I'll have a nervous breakdown,' I said, squeezing his hand.

Danny shook his head knowingly. 'No, you won't. Not now that you're in this hospital where they can prevent that happening.'

I stared at him in surprise. He might just as well have said: You won't have a nervous breakdown now because you're under too much stress.

'But it's *awful* in here, Danny,' I confided. 'I look at patients in OT who are laughing and talking to themselves and ... and I'm scared I might end up like that.'

He frowned. 'Well, look at them and think you're *not* going to end up like that. Be determined not to. Don't give up, Jean. Promise me you'll keep fighting against it.'

Dear Danny. He tried hard to help me. He came to visit me often at first. When he couldn't afford the bus fares, he managed to borrow a pushbike and cycled the seven miles through bitter winter winds to arrive at the hospital, red-faced, hands chapped and numb with cold. He put his beloved guitar aside for a while and got a job in a shop. After finishing work, he'd rush straight to the hospital to arrive promptly at visiting time. Then we would sit holding hands, me falling asleep or withdrawing into a private world of despair – what dismal company I must have been. Danny was a Catholic but he went to a meeting at my old church and talked with Pastor West in an attempt to understand me better.

'All the candles I light at church and the prayers I say are for you,' he said, which reminded me of how selfish my own prayers had become. 'I lit one for you this morning.'

'Thank you,' I said, unable to share his faith but warming a little at the thought of my tiny candle flickering in the cold and darkness of a church, silently testifying that if people care for people, there will always be hope.

*   *   *

I kept careful count of each ECT session, marking the wall behind my bedside cabinet with a pencil. I dressed on Thursday, a morning the ambulance was due to take patients from our ward for ECT, greatly relieved that my course was finished.

'Get undressed! You're having some more shock treatment,' Sister Oldroyd said. Just like that. Not a suggestion but a command.

'I've had eight,' I reminded her.

'Yes, but you're no better.'

I couldn't deny I was no better; I'd never felt worse. But I didn't see how shooting electric currents into my weary brain could help me.

I tentatively asked her why she wanted me to have more and she replied curtly that her reasons were none of my business. Anger broke through my lethargy despite my passive, drugged state. None of my business? It was *my* brain.

'I'm not having any more shock treatments,' I told her. This was my first act of assertiveness in the hospital, my first attempt to gain some control over my life.

'What? Oh yes you are,' she said. The note of confident authority in her voice chilled me. But how could I live with myself if I meekly allowed this to happen?

'No, I'm not,' I said.

She stared at me open-mouthed, then she said angrily, 'You'd better go home then. I've had enough of you.'

'OK. I'll go home.'

'Right. When your parents next visit, let's just see if they'll agree to you going home with them.'

'I'm sure they will,' I said as she walked away. But I wasn't sure of anything. I was trembling at the thought that she might be able to persuade them it would be best if I stayed.

I tried to remember the wording on the ECT consent form I'd signed and realised it hadn't specified how *many* treatments I was agreeing to have. And I remembered Beryl's strange, crooked smile when she'd said, 'Voluntary. Ah, yes. What does that word mean in here?' Well, what *did* it mean? I'd heard others say since that 'voluntary' patients who don't conform to the wishes of the staff could be 'sectioned', in other words detained and treated against their will. Could that happen to me? Could I be forced to have further ECT? My stomach muscles tensed up in a painful spasm; I gripped the bed end. Lord, no!

After breakfast, Dr Sugden arrived on the ward. Since arranging my admission, he had never been to see me, but I gathered he was still ultimately in charge of my treatment. As he was leaving, he nodded to me.

'I'll see you tomorrow,' Dr Sugden said.

I shook my head. 'I'm going home when my parents come this evening.'

He stopped. 'I wouldn't advise that.'

'I don't want more ECT. My parents don't want me to have any more either.' This last bit was added on impulse because I sensed my own views and wishes about my treatment counted least of all. The truth was I didn't know my parents' views about ECT and would have been surprised if they had any. I knew full well they would never have even thought of asking what ECT was and how it was supposed to help me. It wasn't that they didn't care about me but it was just the way they were.

'How many have you had?'

'I was told the course would be six to eight applications and I've had eight.'

'You've had eight?' he asked, stroking his chin.

I nodded. 'And my parents don't want me to have any more,' I said again, remembering that Maria and Tessa, both about my age, said they weren't having ECT because it was against their parents' wishes.

'Well, you're not to have any more, but why this talk about discharging yourself?'

'Sister Oldroyd said I've to go home if I won't have more ECT.'

'I'm sure she didn't say that,' he said, looking at me sternly as if I was a tale-telling schoolgirl.

He called her over and confirmed with her that I'd had eight shock treatments, then he asked if anything had been said to me about having some more.

'Well, Doctor, I did put it to her that perhaps she could be helped by having a few more.'

Sister Oldroyd's mannerism, her tone of voice, everything, was totally different now that she was talking to Dr Sugden. She twisted her fingers, bowed her head and spoke softly. She was deferential, but I realised something else as well. She was scared.

'Did you tell this patient she must have more ECT or go home?'

Sister Oldroyd shook her head. 'Oh no, Doctor, of course not. I merely suggested that more treatment might help, and she flew off the handle.'

'Was anything said about her going home?'

'I only pointed out that we want to help her, and that the sad thing is she might just as well be at home if she won't accept help.'

'I don't want this patient to have more ECT,' Dr Sugden said.

'Yes, Doctor,' she said. Then she turned to me with a sugary smile that was so false it made me want to puke. 'We'd like you to stay here until you get well. You don't have to go home just because you don't want more ECT. Nobody is trying to force you to have ECT, dear. Whatever gave you that idea? You must have misunderstood me.'

'That's not what she said before,' I told Dr Sugden, then I turned to her full of the anger of weeks of bottled-up feelings about the injustice I'd seen and experienced: 'You know very well that I didn't misunderstand you.'

'Hey, that's enough from you!' Dr Sugden said, pointing his finger at me and, with these words, he walked out of the ward and Sister Oldroyd went into her office, leaving me standing there alone with flames of anger burning inside until I could no longer contain them. I rushed to Sister's office, barged in without knocking, and said: 'But you did say I'd to have some more ECT or else go home. You did.'

She was sitting at her desk with her head bent forward and, at my entrance, she looked up, startled. What she said next couldn't have surprised me more than if she had tap-danced on the desk.

'Well, if I did say that,' she said, brushing her fingers across her lined forehead, 'then I apologise. I'm sorry.'

She looked tired and pale. No longer the strict, efficient sister but a woman bending under the burden of a difficult, depressing job. I wondered if she had genuinely wanted to help people at the start of her career, only to become hardened and disillusioned over the years. What was this woman *really* like behind the stern mask? Her apology, if that's what it was, stunned me and I didn't know what to say. In my confusion, I mumbled, 'Well, I'm sorry and I apologise too.'

I left her office not knowing what I had apologised for.

Sitting in the day room, I wondered if I should still try to discharge myself, despite Dr Sugden saying I wasn't to have more ECT. I felt so low I must need help, I thought, though surely not the kind of 'help' offered here. But if I discharged myself, what then? Was she asleep or dead, the girl I'd been before, the girl who laughed and cried and loved the springtime? I think she could have made it. But not now. I'd be an invalid, dependent on my parents, and ... oh God, am I really so sick? What's happened to me?

I was lost in a dark cemetery and too groggy to find my way out, too crushed to motivate myself. As if in some kind of hypnotic trance, I was waiting to be told where to go, what to do. I would stay at the hospital until such time as *they* decided to discharge me. Overcome with fatigue, I lay down on a grave and slept.

CASE NO. 10826

There is really no improvement in this case at all, the girl seems abnormally introverted and withdrawn, is no longer interested in things and is lacking in spontaneity. There is emotional flattening and she herself says I have still got confused thoughts about right and wrong and I do not know who or what I am exactly.

Dr Sugden

CHAPTER SIX

I WASN'T GIVEN ANY more ECT but the heavy drugs treatment continued relentlessly. I, who was once reluctant to take even an aspirin for a headache, now swallowed an assortment of pills three times a day and, despite being almost too sleepy to stand by evening, a sleeping pill each night. From time to time my drugs were changed or given in different combinations though the dulling effects were the same. Pills of all shapes, colours and sizes. Pills with names such as Largactil, Melleril, Haloperidol, Stelazine, Concordin, Mogadon. Pills, pills and more pills. Stupefying drowsiness, dry mouth, shaking body, blurred vision, colossal weight gain, boils like Job's on my chin, neck and chest. It was heavy-handed drugging to the point of brutality. And they called this help, not punishment.

Dull, fogged-up, chemically altered brain, don't give up on me, please. Keep on functioning so that I can think this out and make some kind of sense of it. Lord, I have no strength left to fight any more. I just want to sleep.

But even while stoned on drugs that made me too tired to think clearly, I always remembered to walk away from the medication trolley with my hands unclenched.

'These came for you,' a nurse said, handing me two envelopes when I got back from the OT block one lunchtime. I sat in the day room and opened them. Birthday cards? I'd forgotten.

'I want to die!' shrieked Madeline, curling up on the floor into a ball of noisy tears. Two nurses promptly removed her to give her an injection.

We weren't supposed to show our feelings like that, and I

61

never did. I was crying and dying inside but I just sat quietly. My tongue felt thick, my head fuzzy and I was trying to understand. *Who am I now? My name is Jean. I'm a patient in a mental institution. It's my birthday today. I'm nineteen years old and I wish I'd never been born.*

On the few occasions when Dr Prior talked to me in the Quiet Room, I continued to beg him to lower my medication, but he insisted that the high dosage of drugs was necessary.

'Do you still think about religion?' he asked.

'Yes,' I replied sleepily.

'You do? Oh dear,' he said, tutting and shaking his head gravely as if thinking about religion was a crime. 'I hoped ECT would have wiped it out. We've got to push right down' – he motioned downwards with his hand – 'these thoughts about religion.'

I was sitting opposite him fighting to stay awake enough to take in what he was saying and thinking vaguely that this seemed like brainwashing. I didn't want my thoughts wiped out or pushed down. None of my thoughts about anything. Ever since my first ECT I'd been afraid of forgetting things that were important to me or becoming unable to put them into words. And if, for example, I was to forget for ever, before sorting it out properly in my mind, why the belief about God sending people to hell had troubled me, then ... then I would *never* be whole.

'I mustn't forget anything,' I said.

Dr Prior sighed and wrote something on the papers balanced on his knee while I stared at the floor thinking: They don't understand me. They don't understand me at all.

And I certainly didn't understand the reasoning behind the workings of the system, which had pinned me to the ground, as if beneath big powerful wheels, crushed and broken. If they wanted me to relinquish all thoughts of God, why didn't they try to help me see that life could be bearable, even happy, without a God to believe in? Instead they kept on subjecting me to 'treatment' which made me cry out in desperation to this remote, perhaps fictitious, 'God' to help me. More than ever before I wanted and needed Him now.

I went to a Sunday service at the hospital chapel with Lynette. She didn't like going by herself and I felt I owed her for my passivity during that appalling incident when Sister had been trying to make her eat. It seemed an odd place for a chapel, deep inside the labyrinth of bleak corridors. A large crucifix, above the words 'CHAPEL OF CHRIST THE KING', marked the entrance. A Catholic priest and a Church of England chaplain used this chapel at different times to conduct their services.

The black-robed chaplain took his place at the pulpit and proceeded to lead as 'normal' a service as possible, while an elderly woman seated near the front, her head reverently bowed as if in prayer, was muttering a string of obscenities and meaningless mumbo-jumbo. The chaplain began to speak in what seemed to me like meaningless mumbo-jumbo too. Words fell off his tongue and rolled to the floor.

What was I doing in this chapel? Had I really only come to help Lynette or was I trying to hold on to religion like a drowning person clutches at straws? Hold on. Hold on. No, I have to let go. But, oh dear God, it's hard to face up to being so truly alone in a world that's turned cold and dark and frightening. I can't bear the suffering and sadness I see and feel and breathe in the air all around me.

Tension mounted as part of me struggled to hold on tightly to Christian beliefs while another part was telling me I needed to let go. Hold on. Let go. Hold on. Let go. I didn't even know what I was supposed to be *trying* to do.

Something I remembered reading in the Bible sprang forcefully to my mind: the warning that we ought to fear him who can kill not just the body but the soul. It was not the usual religious meaning of these words that was making the impact. It was the uneasy feeling that this was applicable to the effects on me of the hospital environment and my treatment – that it was destructive not only to my body but also to the very core of my personality, whether one called it the 'soul' or something else. But I must have swallowed the sickness concept along with the pills, for whenever I started thinking and questioning in this way, I would tell myself that this must be the 'sick' part of me, the part I had to 'push right down'.

Push everything right down: bind tears and feelings and questions into strait-jackets. But what happens to all the incarcerated tears? They don't go away. They swell up and multiply inside you, then freeze into blocks of ice. How was I to make sense of these experiences? Was it a dream, a nightmare? No, I really was in a Victorian asylum, along with trapped fish, parched plants, a caged bird and other 'lost' people. I was loaded with drugs and pain. Like the soil in which the potted plants stood, I was cracked and dry.

I began to tend lovingly the wilting, neglected plants that stood on a sill in the day room, watering them daily from a plastic cup. I wanted to make their heads stop drooping so that they wouldn't look like they, too, were drugged senseless. Live and grow; bloom, plants, bloom, and bring some life and colour and beauty to this place of frozen tears.

At Rossfields, my last school, I used to wonder how it would feel if I was at a boarding school or some other place where I'd have to endure my shyness at evenings and weekends as well as through the day. Now I knew.

My three colleagues from work had visited me during the first week of my stay and told me of their great surprise on hearing where I was.

'We'd noticed how you'd always been quiet at work,' Rose had said, 'but we'd no idea that anything was wrong with you. I mean, we thought it was just shyness.'

'But that's right, it was just shyness,' I had said emphatically, though I'd known this couldn't have sounded very convincing in view of my present address.

I realised now that my shyness, confusion about religion, dissatisfaction with my job and social life, letting my family situation get me down, boredom, wondering what life's all

64

about, and other adolescent turmoils, could all be construed through the perspective of psychiatry as symptoms of mental illness. Later, I would think about how this wasn't a constructive way of looking at these kind of problems, and I would wonder why I colluded with the mental health professionals for a long time.

Dr Prior once described me as a 'good patient'. And indeed I was. Good patients believe they are sick and must obey their doctor if they want to get well. Good patients keep on at least trying to believe that the doctor knows what's best for them, even against the evidence of their senses. Good patients co-operate with staff, follow the rules and passively accept their treatment. Yes, I (with the one exception of refusing further ECT) was a very good patient.

Lee's held my job open for as long as possible. I'd worked there for three years since leaving the factory. About three months after my last day at Lee's, my parents brought me a letter at visiting time. It was from Mr Harlow, the Director, asking when I would be returning to work. They had not anticipated such a long absence and were sure I would understand that it was hard for the staff to continue coping with extra work, and temps were expensive. I tried several times to answer this letter, but words wouldn't form on the page; I didn't know what to tell them. I was in the hands of those who were treating me and they never even asked me about my job. I supposed there was no point anyway. My treatment put work out of the question. I asked my father to ring Lee's to tell them I wouldn't be going back.

Mandy visited several times during my stay and she also wrote to me. I was grateful for her reminders of the world outside. Life in an institution – and that's what it was despite any other name they may wish to call it – can be hellish.

I can't make it in this world, I'm simply not going to survive, I thought despairingly, as a dark wave of gloom washed over me, knocking me off balance. I was sitting alone among the crowd of patients in the hall at OT sipping tea from one of the dirty, brown-stained reusable plastic cups. The fact that these cups were never washed adequately had bothered me at first, especially when I watched patients, usually elderly males, using them as an ashtray or spittoon, but now I was past caring. I hadn't seen Raymond for a long time and wondered if he'd cut his wrists again. I looked down at my own white wrists where the veins stood out clearly and knew I hadn't the courage, or whatever it takes, to do it; suicide could never be a way out for me. But how was I to cope with the overwhelming feelings of despair if I couldn't end it all? I couldn't hold on and I couldn't let go. I couldn't live and I couldn't die. Panic gripped my soul. For me, there was no way out.

With my nose pressed to the window pane, I noticed that the white carpet of snow covering the hospital grounds had given way to greenery. Newborn leaves were appearing as tiny shoots on branches of old, gnarled trees. The air smelt of springtime, a season I had once loved. In the mental hospital world it was too easy to lose track of time, but while I was wandering round in a drugged stupor, months were tiptoeing by …

I managed to escape some of the afternoon OT sessions when Dad's friend Joe brought my parents to visit in his car and then took us all out for a ride. On sunny days with the windows open wide we drove down narrow, winding country lanes, past fields, trees and hedges, where the sights and sounds of nature caused a faint stirring within me, a kind of nostalgia for life. It didn't last long. Sister Oldroyd continued to allow Maria and Tessa to go on afternoon car rides with their parents but she told my parents not to visit me in the afternoons because it was causing me to miss OT which was an 'important part' of my treatment.

At OT I fought to keep awake while typing page after page of meaningless prose for copy-typing practice. I had long been a competent typist and at least I'd been paid for doing it at work. When I could bear no longer this 'important part' of my treatment, I would escape to the toilet and allow myself the luxury of drifting off to sleep for a while. I was too drowsy now to write on toilet paper for my diary and, anyway, writing had become as pointless as everything else. But I held on tight to the nostalgia for life that the car journeys had strengthened. In moments of despair I tried to focus my mind on winding country lanes and fields and trees and sunshine till my heart cried out: I want my life back.

Some of the patients were like bloated robots. I looked at them, sadly, and made the connection. I had become just the same. My weight gain was apparently a side effect of at least one of the drugs. I wore long, loose sweaters that hid the large gap where my size 12 skirts wouldn't fasten. Another side effect was that my face and neck kept breaking out in angry, red lumps – far worse than my previous teenage pimples. And Danny had seen me change from the girl he'd known into a lifeless automaton.

When Danny visited I couldn't stop myself from slumping forward and falling asleep at the table where we sat at visiting times. I knew I owed him, and my parents, more than a view of the top of my head when they travelled to see me, but it was so hard to fight against this drowsiness caused by my current dosage of 125 mg of Melleril three times a day, 5 mg of Concordin three times a day and Mogadon every night. I don't think I gave Danny any reason to feel that his visits were worthwhile or that I cared for him at all. On top of this, he'd been putting up with increasing hostility from my father. Danny had told my father he intended to speak to my psychiatrist to query my treatment since its adverse effects were obvious. Dad had told him not to interfere, and couldn't manage even to be civil to Danny after that.

'Jean, wake up and listen to me!' Danny said, one visiting time.

An uncharacteristic tone of agitation in his voice reached my dull senses. I raised my head mechanically and opened my eyes.

'Since you came into this place you've changed beyond recognition and … and I can't stand to see you like this. I'm sorry but I … I just can't.'

'It's OK, Danny, I understand,' I murmured sleepily.

'You want me to go? You want us to finish?'

'Yes. It's for the best,' I said, though I didn't really know what I wanted, except to ease the pain I was causing him and make it easier for him to leave if he wanted to.

A long silence followed.

Finally he said, 'I might go back to Devon, see if I can sort myself out.' His voice was shaky and there were tears in his eyes.

My eyes remained dry; I felt too drugged and distant for tears. I didn't say anything. There seemed nothing left to say.

'Oh God, I ... I'm sorry,' he said standing up. 'I can't bear it any more.'

I followed him to the door of the ward where we kissed goodbye. Suddenly he took hold of me by the shoulders and shook me: 'Please, Jean, don't ...' His voice faltered but his grip on my shoulders tightened till it hurt. 'Don't allow this to happen to you.'

With these words he walked out of the ward and out of my life. I never saw him again.

Jackie visited me just once towards the end of my stay. We'd been friends since primary school but now I felt self-conscious with her, aware of how four months in this institution had taken its toll. She didn't disguise her shock at seeing the pathetic, drugged creature I had become.

'My God, what's happened to you? You're a big fat zombie!' She screwed up her forehead in shocked surprise.

'Let's go sit down,' I said, nodding to the visiting area. Since I'd greeted her at the door of the ward she'd remained standing there, looking reluctant to come right inside.

We went to sit down and she continued to stare at me. 'Your eyes are half closed, your speech and movement is all slow, your body is swollen and your face is so bloated you look like you've got mumps.'

'It's only a temporary thing 'cos of the drugs,' I said, attempting to make light of it.

'But, Jean, I've never seen a person change so much and in such a short time as you have since coming in here. I'm absolutely staggered.'

'Hey, steady on, it's OK, Jackie,' I said, smiling weakly. 'I'm still the same person underneath.' I was desperate to convince myself of that. But I feared I would never be the same again.

And when the transformation was complete; when I had lost my job, my boyfriend, my self-esteem, and had turned into a fat, spotty, zombie-like creature who moved and thought slowly, when I had become withdrawn even with my closest friends (with whom I'd never been shy before), when I felt worse than I had ever felt in my rotten, lousy, fucked-up life and wished I could sleep for ever in a deep, dreamless kind of slumber, they finally decided I was ready to be discharged.

CASE NO. 10826

Progress:
None. There was no essential change in the patient's state in spite of treatment.

Condition on Discharge
Not improved.

Final Diagnosis
Schizophrenia.

Dr Sugden

PART TWO

THE TUNNEL

Selves diminished
 we return
 to a world of narrowed dreams
  piecing together memory fragments
  for the long journey ahead.

Leonard Frank, from 'Aftermath'

CHAPTER SEVEN

I AWOKE AT SEVEN but there was no green light above my bed and no uniformed figures reminding a sleepy ward that it was time to get up. My parents and brother were out, doing their bus-conducting shifts. I turned over, and the next time I awoke it was three in the afternoon. Hunger brought me downstairs just long enough to eat several slices of bread and jam. I swallowed the prescribed dosage of pills, climbed back into bed and pulled the sheets over my head. This is how I spent most of my time during the first days, weeks – how long? – following my discharge.

I couldn't help but reduce my drugs, being often asleep when a dose was due, so gradually their knockout effect eased up a bit. One day while hovering in a twilight world between sleeping and waking I thought about Danny's last words to me: 'Don't allow this to happen to you.' I wondered if I forced myself to go through the motions of living, something might connect and I'd come alive again. With this in mind, I dragged myself into a sitting position, disentangled myself from the dirty, dishevelled sheets and covers, and swung my legs over the side of the bed.

The sight of my dirty arms and legs filled me with repulsion and I was about to go to the bathroom to have the wash I so badly needed when, catching sight of myself in the full-length wardrobe mirror, I gasped. *It wasn't me!* A mental patient wearing my nightgown stared back. She had heavy-lidded, dull eyes set in a bloated face, a floppy fringe and long, straight, greasy hair which hung lankly down to her waist. A big, red lump stood out angrily on her chin and another on her neck.

She was a very fat girl.

I backed away, my face still riveted to the girl in the mirror, then hurriedly pulled open a drawer and fished out a crumpled newspaper cutting of an article I'd written a few months before going into hospital. Below the words '"LET'S BRIDGE THAT AGE GAP" SAYS TEENAGER' there was a photograph of a slim, attractive, smiling teenager with *my* name underneath it. Yes, this was me: the girl in the photograph. And these were my clothes – the size 12 mini-skirts and dresses, which hung lifelessly in the wardrobe, were made to fit a neat, slim figure. I stared back at the fat, ugly girl in the mirror and tears sprang to her eyes.

'That's not me,' I said, wiping my moist eyes on the back of my hand, while the girl in the mirror did likewise. 'That girl who is watching me and mimicking my every movement is not me.'

'I *can't* go out tonight. I look a sight and none of my clothes fit me,' I lamented to my mother as I sat on the settee one Saturday afternoon drying my hair, my old blue dressing-gown pulled tight round my swollen body. In an attempt to rejoin the world of 'normal' teenagers, I'd arranged to meet Mandy that evening.

'Listen, love, why don't you go into town and buy some new clothes?' Mum suggested. 'You can buy a bigger size until your other clothes fit you again.'

Until my other clothes fit me again? I brightened up at the thought that perhaps this fat, ugly, dozy, pathetic creature I was learning to live with had only taken up temporary residence in me. Mum got out her purse and pushed some money into my hand. 'Here, love, take this and go buy yourself summat.'

I went outside feeling like a toad that had crawled out of a hole, blinking uncertainly in the bright sunlight. On the bus I thought the conductor kept staring at me. Had he seen me before and was surprised at how my appearance had changed? Perhaps my brother had told him I was a mental hospital patient. Brian had said everyone working on this bus route knew. Or was I getting paranoid and just imagining the conductor was staring?

In a boutique I tried on a skirt two sizes larger than my normal size but even that was too tight. I'd never before had a weight problem, except for a slight worry that I was too thin. As I returned the skirt to the rack, a young assistant approached me. Her short, psychedelic-patterned mini-dress hugged her sylph-like body and revealed long, slender legs. 'Would you like to try it on?'

'I have done, but it's too tight. I'm just putting it back.'

'The larger sizes are over there,' she said, pointing to the racks cruelly marked 'OUTSIZE'. 'Would you like to look …'

'No, I'll leave it, thank you,' I said abruptly, hurrying from the darkened boutique clutching tightly to remnants of battered vanity. Being fat was a new experience for me.

I went to a large department store and quickly bought a cheap skirt made with ample material and an elasticated waist. I'd always enjoyed buying clothes before, but this shopping expedition was painful. As a reward for getting a tiresome chore over with, I went in the coffee shop and treated myself to a large cream bun, and as soon as I finished eating it I bought another one. Who cared?

I couldn't get too hung up about losing my looks once I got over the initial shock because what worried me most was the death-like change that had taken place on the inside.

No, Dr Sugden, you were wrong to think that there was 'no essential change in the patient's state in spite of treatment'. By the time you were writing this in my case notes I had, indeed, been changed. Wholly and deeply and for ever changed. If the treatment brings greater problems and pain than what is supposedly being treated, isn't there something wrong, Dr Sugden? Isn't there something horribly wrong?

It was hard going out in the evenings again, trying to pick up the threads of my life where I'd left them four months ago. The world of pubs, discos and nightclubs still seemed shallow but I daren't withdraw from the social scene any longer in case I lost touch with my friends. Friends. How precious they were to me. Friends like Mandy and Jackie. How much I needed them. How much I owed them. Without friends, I don't think I could have survived.

Flower Power was still alive in the spring of 1969. Long-haired hippies wearing bells and flowers around their necks pointed the way to a glorious 'alternative' society. It didn't seem as if almost two years had passed since the 'Summer of Love' when Scott Mackenzie topped the charts with 'San Francisco (Be Sure to Wear Flowers in Your Hair)'. Everyone seemed to think this was a wonderful era. Before hospital I'd often failed to see what there was about the sixties to get so excited about, but at least there'd been some fun times too. Not so now. The drugged and electro-shocked me found life more bewildering and depressing than ever.

I tried to tell myself that our generation was lucky to be freed from the sexual hang-ups and inhibitions of previous generations. We could carry a condom in our handbags. Or, better still, take the pill. Have an abortion. Experiment with drugs and blow our minds. Wow! Wasn't it great to be a teenager in the Swinging Sixties? But, having grown world-weary beyond my years, I didn't need to scratch far below the surface to see the pain and sadness beneath the glamour.

Sitting in a pub with Mandy one evening she looked at me sadly and said, 'You're only a shadow of the old Jean I knew.'

'Quite a large shadow though,' I laughed.

Mandy smiled. 'Well, it's good to see you haven't lost your sense of humour. I still keep seeing flashes of that. But tell me what happened. What was it like in the hospital?'

'I didn't exactly enjoy it,' I said flippantly. 'Cor, look at that lad over there. He's dishy, isn't he?'

I didn't want to talk about the hospital, didn't even want to think about it just now. The feeling that I'd been violated and perhaps permanently damaged was more than I could bear.

'I don't understand,' Mandy said. She put down her glass of lager and stared at me. 'You seemed OK until you went in there and then you became all slowed down and it's as if the drugs are draining the life and soul out of you. But what's supposed to be wrong with you? I mean what are they treating?'

'Mental illness, I suppose,' I offered by way of explanation.

'But you're not mentally ill,' Mandy said.

'I think perhaps I am,' I said slowly, tracing the design on a beer mat with my finger. I wondered if this was how members of Alcoholics Anonymous felt when they first publicly admitted to being an alcoholic.

Mandy looked at me long and hard. 'I'll never believe that about you,' she said with feeling. 'Never.'

I don't know if Mandy's faith in my mental health would have wavered if she'd seen me in the café or at the church youth meeting, around this time.

I was eating with my family in a fish and chip café when Brian tried to rope me into a nonsensical argument. I must be crazy, he said, because I'd been in a 'loony bin' so that proved it and everyone he'd told thought so too. When he got tired of the hospital 'digs', he went on to say that I didn't belong in our family and it was time I learnt I wasn't wanted. Throughout the meal he carried on like this while I just continued to eat, quietly listening in my drugged and ECT-induced state of apathy.

Recently Brian had heard me mention to Dad I'd seen Eileen Barrett, a pastor's daughter, in a pub – very unusual for someone from that Pentecostal church. Brian didn't even know Eileen, but after berating me at length for going to dance halls and pubs, he added: 'Eileen Barrett doesn't go in pubs.' I don't know why after not reacting so far to Brian's silly talk, this finally ignited my flattened emotions. I flung the spoonful of sugar I'd been about to put into my coffee across the table into his face, along with the spoon, and shouted: 'YOU'RE FUCKING STUPID!'

The sound of knives and forks scraping plates and the chatter in the café ceased abruptly while people turned and stared.

'Jean, cut that language out!' my mother hissed, her face

77

turning to the colour of the tomato sauce.

'I'll kill you!' Brian said as he tried to get the sugar out of his hair where it had settled like dandruff.

Some elderly ladies a few tables away stared at me in disgust before resuming eating with much tutting, head-shaking and grumbling about not knowing what the world was coming to these days with foul-mouthed young people like me around.

'I'm going now. I've never been so shown up in my life,' Mum said, standing up. 'I'm disgusted with you, Jean.'

'It was Brian's fault,' Dad said. 'I don't know how Jean managed to ignore him for so long.'

But Brian wasn't to blame for the incident at church. This took place one Wednesday evening when nostalgic longing for my old beliefs drew me to the youth meeting. Maybe I was hoping for a miracle to dispel my doubts and make me as happy, innocent and uncomplicated as the teenagers there seemed to be. But when Mr Roberts began talking about God's love, I felt so isolated and pained. No matter how much I wanted to believe, I couldn't help but see countless flaws in Christian beliefs. Unable to contain myself, I interrupted the meeting cutting off Mr Roberts mid-sentence by blurting out: 'IT'S A LOAD OF RUBBISH!'

Heads turned and a moment of uneasy silence followed as in the café. Mr Roberts gave me a quick but searching look. He proceeded to carry on with the meeting but was flustered. I'd once heard him give his testimony saying he used to stammer but God had helped him overcome it. He hadn't stammered for the past thirty years, Praise the Lord, he had said. As he stammered his way through the next few sentences of his talk about God's love I was too embarrassed and ashamed to look at him. Nobody could have been more thankful than me when he managed to regain his composure and normal speech. I had no difficulty in not speaking for the rest of the meeting: I was trying not to cry.

As soon as I could do so without attracting further attention to myself, I left the church and hurried away into the darkness. I roamed the streets aimlessly, thinking about how things at church hadn't changed since I used to enjoy going with Jackie. The church, the preaching and the people were the same. It hadn't made any difference how much I'd wept and struggled and tasted something of a world of despair I barely knew existed before. How could everything else be the same when the sun and moon had fallen out of the sky, plunging my world into darkness? How could everything else be the same when I had changed so much?

Sometimes I wondered if Dad thought about the faith we'd once shared. He'd always said he was leaning on me, but now I didn't feel strong enough to keep myself out of the gutter, never mind lift anyone else out of it. Dad was spending a lot of time with his mate Joe, driving around the red-light areas. He showed me a photo of a teenage prostitute called Nicola lying naked on a bed in a provocative position.

'She tells me she only does it 'cos she needs the money,' he said.

I stared at this photo and wondered if Nicola was happy with her way of life, if she ever had thoughts and feelings and conflicts like mine. Well, why not? We were both products – or victims? – of the same society.

'Dad, do you remember ...' I said, as I handed back the photo. A tear rolled silently down my face. 'Do you remember when we used to pray together?' I caught the tear on my tongue and tasted salt.

'Yes, I remember,' he said, slipping his warm hand into mine and squeezing it tightly. He sighed. 'Something's gone awfully wrong, hasn't it? But yes, Jean, I do still remember.' And there were tears in his eyes, too.

One afternoon when my parents and brother were out on their bus-conducting shifts, Pastor West turned up unexpectedly. I was lying on my bed, zonked out on Melleril. Recognising his car through my bedroom window, I sleepily made my way downstairs to unlock the door. I was wearing grubby pyjamas and my old blue dressing-gown. My hair, in need of washing and combing, hung down in greasy bacon strings. Aware I

79

looked a mess, I could hardly meet his gaze and I was further embarrassed and ashamed by the state of the house, which I had made no effort to clean or tidy.

'Would you like some coffee? I was just going to make some.'

I seemed to be moving, talking and thinking all in slow motion, so I made my coffee extra strong in the hope that it would quickly revive me.

'I'm glad you're out of hospital. How are you feeling?' Pastor West asked as he sat opposite me on a chair from which I'd just hastily removed a pile of old *News of the World* papers.

'Oh, I'm OK. Fine,' I said, not very convincingly. 'Just a bit tired, that's all.'

There was an awkward silence during which I felt he kept staring at me. For the sake of something to say I went across to the mantelpiece and fetched the ceramic tiled ashtray I'd made at OT.

'Look, I made this at the hospital,' I said childishly, pushing it into his hand, like a little girl showing Mummy what she'd made at school.

A mixture of sadness and anger clouded his face as he held the ashtray. 'But this is the kind of thing children make in kindergarten,' he said.

Brian arrived home. He burst into the house, slamming the door shut behind him. When Pastor West had called before, Brian had been either out or upstairs. Today, Pastor West tried to converse with him, just sociable chit chat. When Brian left the room, Pastor West remarked in surprise that he couldn't manage to get anything resembling sensible conversation out of him.

'I know. He's always like that,' I said, fiddling with my hair.

When Pastor West was leaving he stopped at the door. 'I don't know how you can stand it here,' he said. 'You're far more intelligent than your family.'

But not intelligent enough to keep myself away from a mental hospital, I reflected cynically as I watched him drive away. Not intelligent enough to stop myself getting screwed up in the first place. And not intelligent enough to sort myself out now.

Now that I was unemployed, I had each day free to spend as I chose. Ah, strange freedom ... When the drugs wore off a bit, as they inevitably did now that I was taking them less often than prescribed, I sometimes got up before midday and wandered around town. I usually ended up in a dimly lit coffee bar, one of my old haunts, where I would sit for hours thinking. But my thoughts kept bursting like bubbles, then, try as I might, I couldn't remember what I'd just been thinking about.

I did remember, though, that I'd been banned from this place along with Jackie, and two other old school friends, Helen and Kay, because we'd smuggled in a bottle of sherry and were caught drinking it in the Coke glasses. When did that happen? Was it recently or a long time ago? But, anyway, it didn't matter. I had obviously not been recognised now.

At lunchtime, teenagers came and went, put their money into the jukebox, sat in intimate little groups, smoked and chatted. Nobody bothered the girl sitting alone at a table in the corner who was hiding her face behind long, dark hair, slowly sipping her Coke, while Robin Gibb of the Bee Gees kept singing something about being saved by a bell and walking down Heartbreak Lane.

Feeling a need to resort to my old method of catharsis by getting it all down on paper, I bought a thick, ruled exercise book. At night while my family slept, I crept downstairs (my dad would have been angry at me for 'wasting electric') to write at the kitchen table. But how to begin? How many memories had ECT wiped out?

Last week a lad in a pub had said: 'It's me, James! Why are you acting like you don't know me? We said we'd still be friends when we split up.'

'Split up? Did we go out together?'

'Is this some kind of joke, Jean? I don't get it.'

And earlier in the evening Jackie, after recalling times we'd

81

shared, had kept saying in dismay: 'But, Jean, don't you remember when we did this?' I'd thought and thought with increasing distress as I poked inside the cavities in my memory. 'It hurts and scares me when you don't remember these things because they're part of *my* life too,' Jackie had said.

I rested my head on the kitchen table, burying my face in my hands. 'Oh, Jackie, I know what you mean. It hurts and scares me too.'

I searched through last year's diary in which I'd written an entry each day right up to going into hospital on 4 December. I found James in there and, yes, we had dated several times but the memory of him was gone. Robbed from my brain! Horrified, I turned back the pages to January and read on. How strange and frightening it was to read the parts expressing my views on various topics because it now seemed that the author of this diary was someone more intelligent than me. Sometimes I needed to read long sentences several times because I couldn't grasp the meaning or I'd forgotten the beginning of the sentence by the time I got to the end. And all that warmth, passion, youthful idealism; precious parts of myself ... diminished? Gone? Devastated, I mourned the loss of the old me of pre-hospital days. I missed me terribly: it was like a bereavement. Why did they heap stones on my head and bury me alive?

I read on and on until dawn. God, it was painful. Many times I was almost tempted to give up, take my pills and retreat between the bedcovers. But I fought against self-pity and tried hard to force my brain back into functioning properly. I imagined that this was how someone who had sustained head injuries might feel when trying to ascertain how much brain capacity they could hope to regain. But why had they given me ECT? Why had Dr Prior told me there was 'no risk'? Why had no one told me the truth? And, my God, why hadn't I realised myself the inevitable dangers there must be in violently assaulting the brain with electricity? Why the hell had I let them do it?

Morning came and I went back to bed: I hadn't written a thing. I lay in bed watching the shifting shadows of early morning on my bedroom walls. Words kept forming from fragments of thoughts, then teasingly floating away before I could fit them together and hold on to the meaning. My head throbbed with pain as, sick at heart, I grappled with the most distressing question of all. Had ECT *permanently* damaged my brain?

The following night I sneaked downstairs again to sit at the kitchen table with my diaries, pen and notebook. For hours I sat 'looking back' and peering through the fog in my mind at the blank page, until at last it happened: I began writing. Once started, with the aid of my diaries, more memories returned. Throughout the next few nights, I wrote about my childhood and those confusing adolescent years preceding my stay in hospital.

Then I was ready to write about the hospital. Or so I thought. I searched my mind, trying to grasp hold of and fit together my memories of those four hospital months, but I could only achieve something like the fragmented picture of a jigsaw with pieces missing. I was back to staring at a blank page, my stomach knotted with the anxiety of a thwarted need to express my experiences, though the emotional pain was still raw. I had to tell the truth and get it down on paper because what had happened was important and I mustn't ever forget the way that it was.

My head was aching by the time I resumed writing. I pressed on regardless, but the end result was a version of what life in hospital had been like which, although painstakingly accurate, lacked something. I'd always been in touch with my thoughts and feelings (or so I had believed), always been able, at least in retrospect, to lay them on the table in front of me like a pack of cards, to examine, turn over, laugh about, cry about and write about if I chose. But it seemed that the painfully recent memories of those four months in hospital were resisting being pulled out and written about. I wasn't ready to do that. Not yet. Not for a long, long time.

LOOKING BACK 1

HOME FOR MY FIRST seven years was 24 Madras Street in a dingy row of back-to-back houses in Bradford, Yorkshire. An initiation into our rough neighbourhood came when I was only a few weeks old. I was left outside in my pram and a boy thumped me, giving me black eyes.

My first 'cradle' was a drawer from our sideboard. My second bed was a pink cot in which I slept long after I'd outgrown it; I remember having to sleep with knees bent. Brian, my brother, four years older than me, slept in a bed next to the cot. At night Mum would stretch a dark heavy blanket across the window so that the light from the street lamp wouldn't keep us awake (at least I think this was the reason). It made the room pitch dark – perfect for making scary shadows on the walls and ceiling when we became the proud owners of torches. Best of all were the times when Dad came in to kiss us goodnight and he entertained us by making twirly patterns in the dark with two lighted tapers. I would watch, delighted, in childish fascination, as the flames leapt, twirled, joined, separated, like two magical dancers from Fairy Land.

Thick black smoke from the tall mill chimney permeated the air, mingling with the smoke curling upwards from chimneys of houses, and dirtying the washing which hung across the street and in shabby little back yards. We had an outside lavatory inhabited by bluebottles and spiders. Torn pieces of the Daily Mirror hung on a nail inside the rickety door. Rats roamed around the dustbins and Dad said, 'Be careful, Jean, they attack you and go for your throat.'

The area we lived in was known as Little India. Madras

Street led into Calcutta Street and then, a bit further on, Bombay Street was followed by Bengal Street. The air in these streets often seemed to be filled with a strong smell of fried onions that seeped from behind stringy net curtains. Noise never stopped: children yelling, dogs barking, mothers standing on their doorsteps booming out names that often ended on a longer and louder note than the beginning. 'An...DRE E EW!' 'Sus...A A AN!'

Old Mr Benson lived a few streets away and I loved sitting with him on his doorstep. I didn't like the smell of his pipe or his breath but he told me stories and gave me chocolate-covered toffees. He lived near the pub where my granddad used to drink himself into a stupor every weekend. Mum used to say that when she was a girl, if her dad didn't end up lying in a gutter somewhere, she'd hear his foul language as he made his way down Bombay Street, and this was her cue to pull the blankets over her head.

'I knew yer mother when she was nobbut a lass,' Mr Benson told me. 'I remember her coming in The George every Saturday night wearing her Sally Army uniform, a bundle of War Crys under her arm. Such a shy young lass she was. We rough, noisy drunks teased her summat cruel but she kept coming. We asked her to sing. She wouldn't at first. Then one night she stood on a buffet and sang "The Old Rugged Cross". When she'd done you could've heard a pin drop, and then we all started clapping.'

I skipped off home eager to find out more about this.

'Yes, it's true,' Mum said, 'But I daren't go to pubs if yer granddad was there. He'd no time for the Army and he kept threatening to burn me Army bonnet. One day when he was drunk he staggered into a meeting with a cig dangling from his mouth. I was in the songsters at the front. He pointed me out to the whole congregation and announced in a loud slurred voice: "That's my lass there and she's a bloody sight better than all the rest of you lot." I felt awful being shown up like that.'

Dad's parents lived a long walk away from Madras Street, or so it seemed for a child. I didn't see them much. I wasn't close to any of my grandparents. No hugs, no kisses, no sitting on their knees. Years later Dad told me how both sets of grandparents were opposed to my parents marrying 'until I got yer mum pregnant and that changed her parents' tune'.

I was sitting on the kerbside prodding some dirt in a crack in the pavement with a lollipop stick. Not far away lay a dead sparrow. Suddenly I was struck by the force of knowledge that one day my parents would die, I would die, everyone would die. I looked around, half expecting the world to look different in the light of this startling revelation, but, on the line stretched from lamppost to lamppost right across the street, sheets, pillow cases and towels flapped gently in the breeze as on an ordinary day. Did those big girls who were trying to walk with tin cans tied to their feet realise that we'd all be dead one day? Did the boy over there climbing a lamppost know it? Did the two girls who were busily chalking numbers on the pavement for a game of hopscotch? Or that snotty-nosed lad from a few doors on who was throwing stones at a row of milk bottles lined up across our passage? I returned to my dirt-prodding, nursing my grim secret, wondering what death would be like and trying to remember where I'd been before I was born.

But there were plenty of other things to think about in the early morning of my life – such as Santa Claus and bus outings to Blackpool and Easter eggs filled with chocolates.

Next door lived the Bailey kids, Craig and Kevin: leaders of a gang who stomped through the streets chanting in voices loud and proud:

> We won the war
> In nineteen-forty-four

I seem to remember they also had a slogan; I think it was 'STEAL OR STARVE', something like that. You had to step into the gutter to let this gang pass. Winning the war entitled them to take up the whole pavement and not budge for anyone. So big and tough and scary, they demanded respect. Even now it's hard to see them for what they were: just a bunch of ragged, skinny kids. I mean, they must have been. We were all scruffy and hungry. Sometimes the meal of the day was a bag of chips 'with scraps on' from a chip shop called the Wooden Hut.

Craig and Kevin's father, Joe Bailey, was usually singing 'Pack up your troubles in your old kitbag' as he staggered home, but behind closed doors and thin bedroom walls, he unpacked his troubles and slung them at his wife. With each thud from behind the grimy pink roses, I feared that the Baileys would come sailing through and land on my bed. I shuddered, stuck my fingers in my ears and pulled Dad's overcoat, which was used as a blanket, over my head, though I couldn't resist unstopping my ears every now and then to listen to them. 'Don't touch me, yer fuckin' bastard! If yer lay a fuckin' finger on me one more bleedin' time, I'm off ter police, yer fuckin' swine.'

A day or two later Mrs Bailey would emerge with black eyes and bruises. She turned to me, once, as I looked at her with pity. 'An' what d'yer think yer starin' at, yer nosey little bugger!'

Bad language wasn't used in our house then, but I added some colourful words to my vocabulary and was puzzled when told I mustn't use such 'naughty words'.

'But, Mummy, how can words be naughty?'

'You'll understand when you're older,' she said as she put on her long brown coat over her floral pinny. Her thick, chocolate-coloured curls, as always, got flattened when she tied her blue-flowered headsquare tightly under her chin. 'Let's get to the shop before it shuts.'

'Mr and Mrs Bailey don't know they shouldn't say those naughty words,' I said as she buttoned up my warm red coat.

In the corner shop Mrs Bannister weighed our broken biscuits. I could watch her now that I'd grown big enough to see right over the top of the high counter.

'It won't be long afore this whole area's just a pile of rubble,' Mrs Bannister told my mother.

The door pinged as we left the shop. I clutched Mum's hand tightly while we plodded along familiar streets in the flickering lights of the street lamps. Usually I ran ahead with one foot on the pavement and the other foot in the gutter, but this time I kicked a stone and squeezed Mum's hand even tighter. 'Mam, I don't want it to be just a pile of rubble,' I said.

'But we're going to live in a new house,' she said brightly. 'Won't that be nice?'

That night as I lay awake itching with bed bugs and listening to mice scratching, I wove pleasant imaginings of our new house. There'd be no mice in it. It was not that I disliked mice. No, God made 'all creatures great and small' and mice were my friends. I couldn't bear it when my parents caught them in traps. Sometimes they squealed in pain and once, to my horror, I saw a poor creature whimpering around the room dragging its half-severed foot along our brown-patterned lino. My parents said mice spread diseases because they were dirty and, no, we couldn't just wash them.

Each night I added a bit more to this miceless house situated somewhere a million miles away from Madras Street. It would be very big, with lots of rooms to explore. Brian and I would have our own play room stocked with toys, like the little girl in my storybook. There'd be a thick, royal-blue carpet – I couldn't wait to let my bare feet sink into it – and red velvet curtains hanging right down to the floor, and ... I'd been looking through a Home Shopping Catalogue into a different world, and soon I had every room of our new house beautifully furnished and decorated. Then I chose new clothes for us because we couldn't live in such a lovely house and be scruffily dressed as we were now. We'd need swimming costumes, too, of course, to wear when splashing about in the clear blue paddling pool at the centre of our big garden.

Dream on, little girl. Oh, what a pity that reality often does not live up to our hopes or expectations.

CHAPTER EIGHT

I WAS DUE TO attend the psychiatric outpatient clinic at St Luke's on 17 June 1969, about ten weeks after my discharge from High Royds.

'Are you still having problems with religion?' Dr Prior asked, lighting a cigarette and leaning back in his chair.

'Yes,' I said. 'Religion and other things.'

'What other things?'

Ironically, one of the 'other things' was the whole dreadful experience of hospital, but he seemed hardly the right person to understand that.

'My shyness is still a problem,' I said.

I wondered if he realised it was shyness that was making me, even now as I was talking to him, act with nervous gestures and not maintain eye contact. And if he was interpreting signs of shyness as symptoms of illness, did he realise that my social behaviour was quite different with people I knew well?

'Get a book on how to overcome shyness,' he suggested. 'There are plenty on the market.'

We talked next about my need for a meaningful life. At least that's the way I saw it, but when I spoke of feeling restless and unfulfilled, he said, 'I think there could be some underlying sexual frustration.' Trying to discuss my 'identity crisis' brought a similar response.

'I still feel as if I don't know what I am,' I said.

He looked interested. 'Do you mean you don't know whether you're a boy or a girl?'

I shook my head, but he repeated this question at least three times during the interview. I struggled to explain that I meant 'What am I?' not in terms of which sex but something along the lines of: what is a person and what's life all about?

Towards the end of the interview, he chewed his pen. 'I wonder ...' he said, looking thoughtful, 'I wonder if you have a spiritual problem and not a psychiatric problem after all.'

A bit too late for my psychiatrist to be wondering this *after* I'd been hospitalised, drugged, given ECT; gone through the whole machinery of treatment for 'mental illness'... Whether or not it had been a 'psychiatric' problem *before* my admission, I had not emerged unscarred from my journey into the mental hospital world.

I remembered how Dr Prior had pushed the ECT consent form at me while I was too drugged to think straight and how he'd sat with me in the Quiet Room like a cold, unmovable stone while I'd begged him to reduce the drugs when the drowsiness was unbearable.

'I don't understand why I was given ECT,' I said, suppressed anger rising in my throat.

'Well, er ...' He looked down at the notes again. 'You were very quiet and withdrawn in the hospital.'

'Yes,' I agreed, 'but don't you think that could've been partly due to shyness and those drugs? Why didn't you *try* listening to me first instead of drugging me and sending me for shock treatment?'

I sounded accusing, and probably put him on the defensive.

'But you couldn't have talked to me like you have today when I saw you in hospital. That proves the ECT and medication helped.'

It proved no such thing. Dr Prior had only seen me once before getting me to sign the ECT consent form and that was when I was already in hospital, medicated and too tired to talk. Even when I'd first seen Dr Sugden at the outpatient clinic I was groggy with the tranquillisers prescribed by my GP. So neither Dr Sugden nor Dr Prior could possibly compare how I was 'before' and 'after' commencement of treatment. All Dr Prior could compare was how I was 'then' (in the hospital) and 'now'.

'If I was back in hospital now having the same treatment, I'd be just the same as I was then,' I said. But he was reading the notes again instead of listening to me.

'Right, Jean, I'll see you again in a few months. I'm pleased with your progress. Don't you feel you've improved?'

'Well, I have started feeling a bit better since I was discharged,' I said, 'and especially since I reduced the pills.'

'You've done WHAT?' He almost leapt out of his chair, his face changing instantly to a frown. 'Aren't you taking your pills exactly as prescribed?'

'No,' I admitted. 'I'm only taking one dose. At bedtime.'

'Naughty girl!' he exploded. 'If you don't take them properly, you'll end up back in hospital. We don't want that, do we?'

He shook his head gravely, and I shuddered. I hadn't realised the pills were so important. Yet something didn't make sense.

'When I was taking the correct dosage in hospital I'd never felt more depressed,' I pointed out.

'The depression is part of your illness,' he said. It seemed he'd already forgotten that only a few minutes ago he'd been wondering if my problem was 'spiritual' for he was back firmly to the 'illness' definition. 'Now listen to me. It's essential that you comply with the medication. God help you if you slip back!'

Could it really be true that my sanity depended on taking drugs that made me feel so awful? But how come that it was only since treatment had started that I'd been unable to work and began to feel much worse?

'I don't understand,' I said, watching Dr Prior rolling up some papers headed 'History Sheet', his eye on a fly crawling across his desk.

'Well, never mind trying to understand,' he said, swatting the fly with the history sheets.

He looked at me and sighed. 'Just believe what I'm saying,' he said, sweeping his hand in the air as if symbolically sweeping away all the questions that were clamouring about in the part of my brain that was starting to think again. So I was supposed to use blind faith instead of exercising my critical faculties? Wasn't this the same stumbling block upon which lay the weather-beaten remains of my religious beliefs?

'You want to get well, Jean, don't you?'

'Yes, of course,' I said flatly, looking down at my hands resting in my lap. My hands. My lap. Who am I? I am me. What am I? I am me. What is *me*? A naughty girl, a bad child. A mentally ill person who needs mind-bending drugs.

'Promise me you'll take the pills properly.'

I was reluctant to make a promise but the note of urgency in his voice chilled me.

'OK,' I said, feeling scared and confused.

'That's a good girl,' he said. 'I was only angry with you because I want to help you. You do understand that, don't you?'

'Yes. Thank you,' I said quietly, nervously fidgeting and fiddling with my fingers.

He leaned back in his chair balancing it on two legs while staring at me. I felt very uncomfortable with him. The fly that he'd swatted was near the edge of the desk, upturned, crushed and half-dead now: the fragile wings broken but its feet still wriggling.

Starting from when I first saw a psychiatrist, my past was rewritten to fit a 'mental illness' label. No longer a 'normal' teenager with problems but a 'case'. My thoughts and experiences were devalued, their content seen as nothing but 'symptoms'. What little self-confidence I had was crushed out of me. The messages I received were loud and clear: I would never be a writer; never amount to anything much. Something was fundamentally wrong with me; my brain needed changing. I was tragically flawed. If I couldn't believe this, it meant I lacked what psychiatrists define as 'insight', that I was so sick I didn't even know I was sick. With hindsight it's obvious that I should have stopped complying. But the vulnerable, naïve teenage me at the time was frightened into trying to be a 'good girl' by Dr Prior's warning about going back into hospital if I didn't take my medication. I threw away my correspondence course lessons in Journalism which I'd been hoping to resume, if only as a hobby, suppressed my questions, swallowed my pills – and spent most of each day sleeping my life away.

About a month after Dr Prior had scared me into resuming the full medication, I vaguely remember Dad waking me to tell me I was missing the moon landing. Did he think I gave a toss that a man was walking on the surface of the moon? I turned over and went straight back to sleep.

I could drift along for a while feeling too tired to think, too sick to care, but every so often I did wonder how and when this was going to end. Before hospital, getting a bed-sit and a more interesting job had been important to me, but now just getting *any* job seemed out of reach. And jobless, drowsy and depressed, how could I get somewhere suitable to live? How could I begin to carve out some kind of a life for myself? I knew I must fight harder against this weariness, these feelings of despair; this strange and terrible sickness that had laid me low.

'Jean, you *have* to get well,' I mumbled, tensing up my body and gripping my pillow tightly. But knowing no way I could achieve this elusive state of being 'well', and feeling achingly empty and low, I reached for my pills and escaped again in sleep.

So how was this happening? How could I be up on the stage at the Mecca telling hundreds of people which outfits I thought would suit Twiggy? No, it wasn't a dream. I really was reading into a microphone the words I'd scribbled earlier on to a slip of paper. Words written when, on arriving at the dance hall, Mandy and I found everyone entering a competition. Simple. All we had to do was look at the clothes being showcased in the foyer from a local boutique and 'choose the two items you think will look great on Twiggy'.

Out of all the entry slips that could have been picked out, I was the 'unlucky' winner. When they called my name, I wanted to run out of the door instead of walking up on stage. If it hadn't been for Mandy I wouldn't have admitted the name belonged to me. But Mandy waved her arms about excitedly. 'Go on, Jean. You've won.'

It was just a raffle really. I hadn't won because of the wisdom of my words, that was for sure.

'I think outfits numbers two and four will best suit Twiggy …' The microphone crackled. '… best suit Twiggy because she's slim and these will look good on someone as slim as her.'

Oh, God, did I really write this crap?

After reading out my piece, I still wasn't off the hook yet.

'And what do you think of Twiggy?'

Twiggy. 'The Face' of the sixties. What did I think of her? What did I think of *anything* with my mind shot to pieces? I stood, self-consciously in the spotlight, and prayed I would pass for normal.

'She's … er, she's nice.'

'Well, let's give a big round of applause for the lucky winner of our competition who'll be coming to Bo's Boutique to choose one of these gorgeous outfits.'

Everyone clapped me back to my seat. I just wanted to fade away into insignificance again.

One of the ironies of being on drugs is that the treatment for side effects involves prescriptions for yet more drugs. In hospital many of us suffered from constipation as a result of drug treatment, for which we were given regular doses of laxatives. I was also prescribed, later, a drug to help alleviate the side effects of neuroleptic drugs, such as the Parkinson-like tremors. For the ugly, big lumps that kept erupting on my face and neck, Dr Prior referred me to a dermatologist who diagnosed 'adolescent acne', prescribed a course of x-ray treatment and yet more drugs.

It seems, however, that I was now on a different drug from that which caused the enormous weight gain in hospital, or else my body must have made some adjustment to it, because I was much less bloated. Although my face without make-up remained extremely pale with a yellowish tinge and my eyelids still drooped heavily over dull, tired eyes, I must have looked at least presentable because boys started taking an interest in me again. In fact, I was never short of boyfriends despite, or perhaps because of, my lack of interest in them. Mandy said it must be that I presented a kind of challenge to them because most other girls were keen to have boyfriends and then to get married, but I was different.

'No, it's not that I don't want to get married,' I tried to explain to Mandy. 'If I fell in love, then I probably would want to get married, but the lads I meet just don't interest me.'

'Well, who would?' Mandy asked. 'Do you think you're somehow special, different, from us lower mortals?'

'Heck, no!' I said, feeling uncomfortable. 'It's just that I don't want the kind of life that … that most people settle for.'

'Well, what sort of fella do you want to meet? What kind of life do you want? What else is there?'

I smiled wryly. How often had I asked myself these same questions. Ironically, it seemed that in wanting more out of life than most girls, especially working-class girls like myself appeared to want, I was in great danger of ending up with much less.

Coming home from a pub with Mandy one night, we watched a woman lurching along the pavement in front of us. She was a pathetic creature, shabbily dressed, hair matted with dirt, and she stank to high heaven of whisky mingled with the diarrhoea that stained the back of her dress, the urine that trickled down her legs and the vomit that dribbled from her chin. Who was she? Perhaps somebody's mother? Somebody's wife? Somebody's daughter, certainly. She had been a child once. What had brought her to this? Where did she live? Had she anywhere to sleep tonight? Did anyone care?

Mandy nudged me and pulled a face. 'Now, isn't that the most disgusting apology for a person you ever did see in your life?'

But I was thinking of one of my favourite songs on my Joan

Baez LP, and never before had the words 'There but for fortune...' seemed more hauntingly, poignantly, frighteningly true.

I wished I could reach out to her, help her in some way. But what could I do? Then my thoughts took a more selfish turn.

'I hope I won't end up like that,' I whispered.

'What?' Mandy turned to me in astonishment. 'Jean, how can you even think of saying such a thing?'

This pulled me up sharply. I hadn't realised it would seem to Mandy such an odd thing to say. Not long ago, I would have observed from a safe distance, unaware of the slightest possibility that I might one day end up without pride or decency like this wretched woman. But it didn't seem impossible when viewed from the tunnel.

Cold, black tunnel days. Days when I slept my time away. Days when a soul-aching darkness engulfed me and sucked me into a void. And days when I switched on to 'automatic pilot' behaving like a zombie that had been programmed to make 'appropriate' responses. There were times when I feared I might make a crash landing and break into pieces that would be scraped up from the ground, bottled, corked, labelled and stored away in High Royds where nobody would notice that somewhere pushed down underneath a drugged haze there was a real person; somewhere there was JEAN.

Often my 'automatic pilot' didn't work properly, allowing my old questions and confusion to infiltrate, such as when I was dancing with mock carefree abandon at a disco one weekend and found I couldn't turn off the question: What kind of life *do* I want? I only knew what I did *not* want. I did not want the TV and bingo life of my parents. I did not want the life of the other teenagers in this place. And I definitely did not want the kind of life I was living. If this was all there was, then why bother to breathe?

It was two in the morning and I hated his kisses. I pulled away and pushed through the crowd of sweaty bodies to the edge of the dance floor. The heat was stifling and my throat felt sore with the cigarette smoke which clouded the place.

I leant against the cold, stone wall near where a long-haired, bearded youth, wearing torn blue jeans and a T-shirt displaying a big 'FREE LOVE' badge, was lying on the floor dead to the world. I watched his long, matted hair change colour in the flashing lights – now green, now orange, now purple – and I wondered if he was happy. I was always wondering that. I could not accept that I alone was acting and that other people were happy with this farce called life.

Those feelings of despair again ... I felt like a prisoner longing for a glimpse of the sun.

'I don't belong here. I can't bear this life. Lord, get me out of this, help me please.' No answer. Nothing. Just lights flashing in darkness and a young woman scantily dressed in a leopard skin dancing in a cage above a platform where a shaggy-haired, guitar-twanging pop group were belting out something about 'lurrrve' to a hot, sticky mass of gyrating bodies on the dance floor.

'Wanna dance?'

Our bodies moved to the rhythm of the music. His lips pressed against mine and I felt his tongue in my mouth as his hands wandered over my body. 'Lord, help me,' I was still praying. 'I can't live this way.' But I was kissing him too.

'Great place this, ain't it?' he said.

I nodded.

'Enjoying yourself?'

'Yeah, sure,' I lied.

'Wanna drink?'

I downed it quickly. A double vodka this time. Drinks helped me to act. I was a pretty good actress by now but I wanted out. I was sick to death and wanted to quit the whole damn show. But I didn't know how. What else was there?

He slid his hand up my leg under my mini-skirt and fumbled about. At first I made some feeble attempt to push him away so that I could cling to some shreds of self-respect, but I was so tired; I didn't even know what I was supposed to be fighting against any more. I remembered Mr Roberts, Youth

Leader at church, saying 'It's easiest just to go along with the crowd. After all, a dead fish floats downstream.' But nobody had ever told me that dying fish cry and ache and hurt deep down inside as they feel themselves losing the battle to muster enough strength to turn and swim against the tide.

We sat on the floor near the wall and I leant against his shoulder. Stoned on a mixture of drink and medication, I kept drifting in and out of sleep but I was aware of his hand under my blouse and I kept waking when he squeezed my breast so hard that it hurt.

'Let's dance again,' I said, disentangling myself from him and pulling him to his feet.

I tottered towards the dance floor, feeling as if I was walking in a dream and nothing was real. Pop records were belting out and I managed to give myself up to the noisy music and wild disco-dancing, my waist-length hair flying about in all directions.

How long can a person go on separating their real feelings from their actions? Acting, pretending. Knowing full well it can only be leading to self-destruction. Being vividly aware of something does not always shed light on the solution, and I could see no way out, didn't know what I should be doing and felt utterly lost and confused about life. So the show went on.

And there was my family situation too. Tap. Tap. Tap.

'Shut up, Brian.' A foolish grin. More taps. Coins now: that infernal clinking sound. Prods. Digs. Mustn't lose my temper, it would only worsen the situation. Pretend I don't care. Pretend to be reading a magazine. Hum a tune as if happy. Yes, I could carry it off. I was awfully good at pretending with all the practice I'd had. But still the clinking, the tapping, the silly talking. Why? For God's sake, why?

'Bloody shut up!' I exploded, finally allowing my bottled-up feelings an outlet.

'Now cut that language out, Jean. If you can't control your tongue, you can't control anything,' Mum said.

More clinking. Louder and louder.

'If he doesn't bloody shut up I'll kill him!' I shouted.

'Take your pills,' Mum said, handing the bottle to me.

'Yeah, take your pills, Jean,' Brian said with a grin.

'I don't want them. It's you lot who's sick.'

'Nobody in this family has been in a mental hospital except for you, so don't insult us,' Mum said indignantly. 'Take your pills and go to bed.'

Well, there was some temptation to do that anyway. So I swallowed several pills and went to bed.

Oblivion. Peace of sorts. Until I awoke …

Bright light hurting my eyes. Sunshine. Daytime? It must be. The sound of an ice-cream van. Children playing outside. More sleep. Darkness. Middle of the night now. More sleep. More pills. Pills and sleep and day and night all mixed together in darkness and confusion. A living death. I used to be happy once. I think I did. What went wrong? Jesus, am I sad or bad or mad?

Church bells ringing. It must be Sunday. Memories of childhood Sundays and childhood schooldays. Shifting myself up into a sitting position I slumped forwards with head in hands before crawling groggily out of bed. I washed my face, put on my old jeans with a crumpled T-shirt, hungrily devoured several slices of toast and gulped down a mug of strong coffee. Then, still feeling like death, I went outside to roam the streets searching for I knew not what. My lost childhood perhaps.

I wandered into the playground of Drake Street Junior School and peeped through the window of my old classroom. How small those desks and chairs were. I pictured a classroom scene from years ago. Christmas in the late 1950s. Bright coloured balloons and paper chains decking the walls. Sylvia and I, aged about eight or nine, sitting there at that desk in the front row, eyes and minds agog as our teacher, Mr Hales, read extracts from *A Christmas Carol*. And I remembered how vividly I'd imagined Scrooge peeping through the window into his old classroom, looking with wistful longing at the child he had once been. Today I was the person looking through the window with the Ghost of Christmas Past at my shoulder.

Before leaving the schoolyard I went to look at the toilets with their funny low pots. Had they *always* been so small? I wandered back out of the old school gates and down the road, stopping outside the Salvation Army to listen to the singing.

I crept inside the Army hall and sat on the end of the back row, remembering a time long ago when life, including religion, was simple. And then back home to more pills, more sleep.

LOOKING BACK 2

THE MAN WITH SLICKED-BACK, greasy hair was up to no good. You could tell that by the way he leered at the woman in the white cardigan. She was strolling along the quiet, leafy footpath. A twig cracked under his foot. 'Behind the tree,' I whispered, to warn her. Nervous glances over her shoulder. He quickened his pace. His hand reached down into his overcoat pocket. Close behind her now. I strained my eyes to see what he was twisting around his fingers. A piece of rope. And then...

Blackness.

'Oh, blow! Where's me purse?' Mum said.

We stared in dismay at a tiny, fading spot of light in the centre of a black screen. 'I told yer to check the meter before it started,' Dad said.

Mum groped her way out of the room to feed the hungry electricity meter. By the time the telly came back on, the credits were going up. This happened often. Without warning, we'd be plunged into darkness at the part in the late-night thriller where the heroine was about to be strangled, the goody was about to be shot or the snake was slithering up the leg of the cot. 'We've gotta make sure the meter's full before we start watching owt,' one of us would say.

Apart from those late-night horror films, I loved watching Robin Hood starring Richard Greene. Another favourite was Popeye the Sailor Man who could suddenly turn from a weedy wimp into a fearsome fighter of bullies just by eating a tin of spinach. I pestered Mum to buy me spinach, something I'd never heard of before.

Madras Street had been demolished as part of a slum

clearance plan when I was seven. We'd moved to 40 Spring View, a house on a recently-built council estate. Our new house had no play room, no red velvet curtains and no big garden with that clear-blue paddling pool of my dreams. But we had got an indoor toilet, a bathroom, and electric lights. Better still, Brian and I had separate bedrooms. And then we got the telly. We had become posh.

I made five 'best' friends in my new class at school: Shirley, Sylvia, Carrie, Julia and Jackie. All of us, except Jackie, lived in Spring View, so I always had someone to play with.

My friends and I would set off early in the morning on Saturdays or school holidays, carrying jam sandwiches wrapped in paper and wearing plastic water containers round our necks. We walked miles down Wagon Lane, a pebbly dirt track, leading to swampy pools, stretches of wasteland and a wood; an area we called Rainbow Land. Unaware of the real dangers of such a lonely place, our imagination transformed the area into a perilous jungle, an enchanted forest or an island in paradise.

Mum had a full-time job in a mill now and Dad still worked on the buses, while I enjoyed school holidays unsupervised from an early age. Three of my friends were in one-parent families with a working parent. The way we roamed freely must seem strange today but it wasn't unusual for a lot of children then. We didn't have watches and often only knew it was time to head back home when we became tired and hungry.

The pockets of my old blue jeans bulged with tubes of fruit gums, Swizzels, and the like, as we strolled down Wagon Lane. My friends, too, had knobbly bits caused by pockets full of sweets bought after saving up spending money. We shared them out to get a good mixture. 'A green fruit gum for a pink loveheart? Not a black fruit gum; they're worth at least three lovehearts.' 'Only a few Swizzels for a gobstopper? No, get lost!' 'Oh come on, Carrie, one of my flying saucers with sherbet inside has to be worth more than a lemon Opal Fruit.' (Even our squabbles were fun.)

Jeans or shorts with bright-coloured T-shirts, and grey plimsolls that had started life white, were my typical Rainbow Land clothes. A casual green corduroy jacket sufficed for the cooler days of which there seemed only a few. It never rained there. No, that can't be true. Wasn't that the place where the biggest and best rainbow I'd ever seen in my life decorated the sky? It must have rained. I can't remember.

From the ages of about eight to twelve, we spent long summer days in Rainbow Land. We rarely saw anyone else there. This was our place where we were free to live and grow. We climbed trees, drew pictures, sang, danced, wrote stories and poems. We also wrote plays which we acted out. And we couldn't have been happier feasting on delicacies at some picturesque beauty spot than we were, sitting among weeds, eating jam sandwiches.

One sunny day in Rainbow Land, I was sitting with Carrie under the outspread branches of a great oak tree. We were both aged nine. She looked up from the picture she was sketching and asked, 'D'yer have a secret dream, Jean, summat you most wanna do when you grow up?'

'Tell me yours and I'll tell you mine,' I said.

'OK. But promise not to laugh.'

'I won't laugh, cross me heart.'

We lay on our backs in the long grass. The sun was making moving criss-cross patterns through the leaves on our arms and legs. I shut my eyes and could still see them.

'I wanna go to Art School when I grow up,' Carrie said. 'I showed Dad some of me pictures yesterday and he said they're good. He said maybe I'll be able to go to Art School.'

I rolled on to my stomach and picked at the grass. 'When I grow up I wanna be an author. I mean a proper one, and get stories and books published.'

'We could do it together. You write the stories and I'll draw the pictures.'

Jesus was very real to me in those Rainbow Land days. As real as sunshine and dewdrops and woods full of bluebells. Mum hadn't worn the Salvation Army uniform for many years, but Brian and I did; he was in the Junior Band and on my eighth birthday I became old enough to join the Singing Company. If there's one thing I cannot and never could do it's sing in tune. My school teachers knew better than to let me into the school choir, but my wonderful Sunday school teachers must have interpreted 'Make a joyful noise unto the Lord' to mean something even a frog could do.

Sunday was The Lord's Day. It started with the junior meeting at 10 a.m. after which Brian rode home on his bike, while I caught the bus. Often, by the time I arrived home, Brian was eating his last mouthful of beans on toast or fish fingers from the plate on his knee. The afternoon junior meeting started at 2 p.m., followed by the adult meeting from 3 p.m. to 4 p.m., which my parents sometimes attended.

We clapped and sang rousing songs as the band played and tambourines danced in the air, their coloured ribbons flying. A short, fat man with a shiny bald head sat in the front row of the band, blowing an enormous trumpet. As I watched his puffed-out cheeks growing redder, I imagined him bursting with a loud bang and ending up in red rubbery pieces like my balloon.

For the boring parts of the adult meetings, I invented a game. Timing myself with the second-hand of the big clock on the wall, I practised holding my breath for as long as I could in an attempt to beat my own record. My talent for this improved tremendously during one meeting when a long-winded speaker droned on. But this was the last time I played this game. The 'Jesus Saves' slogan, which was painted in large black letters beneath the Army crest on the wall, began to dance and spin dizzily. I gasped, and almost passed out.

It was never boring with Captain Ann Costello. In one of the meetings she pulled a mat onto the platform, slipped out of her shoes and bonnet, and did a lively song and dance routine, acting out the parts of David and Goliath alternately. The grand finale was when she ended up as the dead giant lying flat on her back, staring wide-eyed at the ceiling.

I was proud to wear the Singing Company uniform of navy skirt, white blouse, red tie, and navy beret with the Army crest, However, I did occasionally hide in a passage to take off my tie and beret before hurrying past gangs of lads on my way from the meeting to the bus stop.

Ashamed of myself for this cowardice, I decided one day to face the den of lions in my uniform. I hoped to slip by unnoticed but one of the lads pointed at me and yelled, 'Look at her! Sally Army!' About eight pairs of eyes were on me. I held my head high and strode along boldly, trying to hide my nervousness. The knot of tension in my stomach tightened even more when they all closed in on me. They began chanting familiar lines:

> Salvation Army free from sin
> All went to heaven in a corned beef tin.
> The corned beef tin was much too small.
> They all fell out and the devil got 'em all.

But that was it. I'd got off lightly. Jesus had protected me.

I was still young enough to believe all I was taught at Sunday school. Many of my favourite songs were in my starcard, the children's slim songbook stamped with stars denoting our attendance. Mention of hell didn't bother me. I wasn't questioning then how a loving God could send anyone to suffer in torment for all eternity. All they had to do was ask Jesus to come into their hearts. I was safely protected by the simplicity of a child's mind from the deeper complexities of religious belief, of death, of life.

> Gentle Jesus, meek and mild,
> Look upon a little child;
> Pity my simplicity,
> Suffer me to come to Thee.

Throughout the years of my childhood I said these words in prayer each night. Throughout the years of my teens I looked

105

back with a wistful longing for that simplicity which I had lost.
Pity my simplicity. Pity?

CHAPTER NINE

IN THE WASTELAND OF the days following my stay in hospital, how I wished I could return to the 'pity my simplicity' days of childhood. Dear God, I had come a long way since then.

Must get up now to meet my friends for another evening at the pub. I crawled out of bed in the early evening and put on my lime-green mini-dress that zipped up the front from neck to hem. No, not a good idea. Gropers were keen on that dress. I changed into my cream flared trousers and a psychedelic-patterned tunic top, my prize from Bo's Boutique for winning the Twiggy competition. No, too gaudy and snazzy. Didn't feel right somehow. Try again. I got into my old pair of denim jeans and a grey-checked shirt-style blouse. Yes, that would do. I used to enjoy shopping for clothes but since the hospital I couldn't be bothered. Anyway, a pair of old jeans and a few non-iron tops were all I needed.

My long, straight hair required minimal attention. All I had to do was attack my fringe with the kitchen scissors each time it grew long enough to make me cross-eyed. Lopping a lot off it that night made my dull, tired eyes show up. On with the dark-grey eyeliner and brownish-black lash-thickening mascara. 'Oh well, better to look made up than drugged up,' I said to myself, staring in the mirror. Trouble was I looked both. But in the dimly lit pub it didn't matter.

Drinks. Laughter. False gaiety masking the tears inside. Mustn't let anyone know. Got to hold myself together, face the world, and pass for 'normal'. Who keeps putting 'Behind a Painted Smile' on the jukebox?

More drinks. More laughter. Have another gin. And another.

See how it sparkles in the glass. Looks pure and clean as spring water. Goes down more easily than pills too. In the purple shades of evening I made my way home past street lamps that wobbled on pavements that tilted.

Mum and Brian were at work. Dad was asleep on the sofa when I arrived home. He woke when I gave a loud hiccup.

'Why haven't you got a job?' he demanded.

I shrugged my shoulders and giggled, then I stumbled into the bathroom to clean my teeth. Dad came in and dragged me away from the washbasin, knocking the toothbrush from my hand. I was gagging on a mouthful of frothy, minty toothpaste as he made me go to bed.

'Tomorrow you get a job,' he said firmly.

Toothpaste and gin. Headache and nausea. The room spinning. I'm falling down, down, down into darkness ...

I must have been asleep for a few hours but it seemed like only minutes before I heard my father's voice again.

'You get up now, do you hear?' He flung off the covers and tugged roughly at my arm. I glanced at the clock. Four in the morning. I dressed quickly and sat, shivering, in the kitchen.

'Go out and get a job,' Dad said, glaring at me fiercely, as if he expected me to do so that very minute.

'I can't at this time of the morning, can I?' I said this timidly, not defiantly; his moods could still frighten me.

'Well, if I come home from work and find you in your pyjamas again I'll kill you. When the Sister at High Royds told me you were in need of discipline, I couldn't understand it because –'

'What? She told you that?'

'Yes, when I came one visiting time. I couldn't understand it then because it was Brian, not you, who needed discipline, but I won't put up with the way you behave now. You grumble about the state of the house but you don't lift a finger to clean it. Lazing in bed all day, staying out late at nights, coming in drunk. Well, I'm not having it any more. The first thing you'll do is get a job and start earning your keep. Do you hear?'

I stared at some crumbs on the faded brown lino.

'I said, do you hear?' he shouted, his lips close to my ear. My aching head reverberated with sound.

'Yes,' I said quietly. 'I hear.'

When he'd set off for work, Mum came into the room, and I vented my feelings on her.

'He drags me out of bed at four in the morning and tells me to get a job,' I grumbled.

'Well, you should try to be sensible.'

'Where did trying to be fucking sensible get me?'

'You should cut out that disgusting language, and you shouldn't have come home drunk last night.'

'Anyway, I'm supposed to be sick. If I'm treated like I'm sick in the head, then why shouldn't I act like it?'

'You should go to bed early at night, then you'd get up early next day. And you should take your pills.'

'I *do* take the flaming pills. That's why I'm always either asleep or wandering about like a zombie. I might as well be dead.'

'You *are* dead. Dead in trespasses and sins.'

'Don't talk so fucking stupid! Why can't you try to understand?'

'I *do* understand. You know yourself what you really need. You ought to go back to church.'

'You don't understand anything,' I said.

But I was thinking: And neither do I.

A cold, damp evening a few months later. Brian and Dad were on late shifts. I was staying in with Mum. She sat reading a magazine. Disturbing images filled the TV screen. I watched, transfixed, and then I began scribbling some thoughts on to paper.

> *Television brings news and documentaries about human misery into the comfort of our living rooms. I can watch people dying in Vietnam, and right here in the corner of my room, starving children in Biafra rub their bone-thin fingers over grotesquely swollen bellies while I'm eating*

my tea and counting the calories. Not one of these children (who have never really been children) will even have the chance to grow up into a confused, cynical adolescent like me with time to bother about the meaning of life. As soon as the television is switched off, it's easy for us well-fed English teenagers to forget about what's going on in faraway places, as long as we drop a coin in a collecting tin every now and then, and proudly display our 'MAKE LOVE, NOT WAR' badges. And yet what can I do anyway? Why doesn't He who promised to feed even the sparrows help them?

The sharp ringing of the phone broke into my thoughts. Mum jumped up and rushed to answer it as if she'd been waiting for a call.

'What? *Now?*' Mum asked with a giggle. 'Well, I suppose I could do. Yes, OK then.'

She giggled again, twisting the telephone wire round her finger. I picked up her discarded magazine and pretended to read. More girlish giggling. When she put the phone down she rummaged in a drawer and pulled out her make-up and blonde wig.

'Are you going out?' I asked in mock surprise.

'I might do.'

'Oh? Ten minutes ago you said you were going to have a bath and an early night,' I reminded her.

'I might happen to change my mind.'

'Call me and I'll come running. So you're off to meet your fancy man?'

She was having an affair with Roy, a bus conductor in his twenties. Almost young enough to be *my* boyfriend.

'What I do is my business. I'll mind my business and you mind yours, Lady Jane.'

'That lipstick looks awful,' I told her.

She pulled the blonde wig over her straggly, greasy hair which was once a rich, dark brown, now heavily sprinkled with grey.

'If you must wear a wig why don't you buy one that at least looks like *real* hair? And why blonde? It doesn't suit your complexion.'

She changed into a short skirt.

'Cor, talk about mutton dressing up as lamb,' I commented.

The front door banged and I listened to the sound of her high-heeled shoes as they clicked along the pavement.

'You're a cheap tart!' I yelled at the closed door.

What a fool she was making of herself. Oh, if only I had sensible parents, I thought, then maybe I, and even Brian, would have turned out all right.

I pulled on a thick woollen jumper over my faded blue jeans, grabbed my jacket and left the house. I was determined not to go back that night. Let Mum worry about me. Serve her right. 'I must ditch the self-pity and stop blaming others', I had written in my diary only the previous evening. But I was sick of trying, sick of everything.

I caught a bus into town and wandered the streets aimlessly before heading for the Big Sound, an all-night disco. It'll be safer and warmer to spend the night in a disco than out on the street, I thought decisively, turning up my collar against a chilling breeze and the first spots of rain. But the thought of the ear-splitting music, the dismal, smoky atmosphere, the sweaty bodies packed together like sardines in the dark and, worst of all, the endless ritual of kissing and petting with lads I neither knew nor liked, nauseated me. I stopped and leant against a wall to think things over. I didn't want that way of life. Not tonight. Nor any other night.

I roamed the streets for what seemed ages; head down, staring at pavements shiny with rain. The town hall clock struck eleven. I had an idea. My last bus was due to leave town in fifteen minutes. I would be on that bus. But I wouldn't be going home.

Sitting on the smoky top deck watching the heavily made-up wives with their red-faced boozed-up husbands and eavesdropping on their meaningless talk, I felt more and more isolated. Surely people were meant for better things, yet what

111

'things'? Supposing those religious experiences, which had seemed so wonderful, if only for a short time, had awakened in me a craving for 'spirituality' that would never subside, leaving me destined forever to be disillusioned with the world?

Now that I'd no longer got my pie-in-the-sky-when-we-die beliefs to make it more palatable, I still had to live in this rotten, lousy world that I didn't feel at home in. One glimpse of heaven for the price of hell!

'Fares please!' said the conductor, jolting me back from the edge of the abyss.

Force of habit almost made me stand as we neared the stop where I usually got off. But as I gazed through the rain-splattered bus window at our house, all I could think was I didn't want to go home. More than anything else I didn't want to go home.

At the terminus I pretended to adjust my shoe until the other passengers had gone, then I tiptoed to a seat near the front and crouched. I listened anxiously as the conductor climbed the stairs and walked along the aisle sliding windows shut. His footsteps grew nearer but then, to my relief, I heard him going back down the stairs. The lights were turned off and the bus, with its stowaway, sped towards the depot.

The bus stopped with the engine still running. Then it started moving again. Slowly, and from all sides, came swishing, thumping, rubbing sounds with a closing in of something dark green. 'Help, what's happening?' I whispered, gripping the metal handrail on top of the backrest of the seat in front, but it was only the large, mechanical bus washers. At last the bus was parked for the night. The driver and conductor whistled and chatted as they walked away.

An eerie silence descended over the lingering smells of the engine and stale cigarette smoke. Peering through the windows I saw that my bus was flanked on either side by two empty buses. I stretched my legs, moved into a more comfortable position – and began to wonder what the hell I was doing alone on a cold, dark bus in the middle of the night.

Then the thoughts really started. First, about High Royds; a painful reliving of those four months. And then about the church beliefs. Could anything be worse than living for ever and ever with no hope of annihilation?

'God, how can you be so cruel?' I whispered accusingly. 'Why can't non-Christians cease to exist when they die? What kind of God are you? Sadistic? Oh, I ...' But I stopped short of saying, 'I hate you.'

I tried again: 'Jesus, I don't understand. I don't understand anything.'

Humbled, I was praying in a different vein now. 'Help me get through this difficult stage of my life.'

But the more I tried to invoke the intervention of God with my last remaining grains of faith, the more the conflict intensified. I sank to my knees, my face buried in the bus seat, cold beads of perspiration sticking my fringe to my forehead. 'Please help me, God, if you are there. Oh, please still this storm inside of me ... It's tearing me apart.'

Just look at you, Jean, I said to myself as if observing coolly from a distance. A weak, snivelling wretch who is looking for easy answers. You still haven't let go. What do you expect now? An Angel of Light to appear?

No, no, there is no God to help me and no Satan to hinder me; that's just superstitious mumbo-jumbo.

Yes, but the conflict in your mind indicates you're mentally sick, Jean. If a psychiatrist could see you now, you'd be taken straight back to High Royds.

No. No. It can't happen to me.

Oh, can't it? Of course it can. Plenty of other people have gone crazy and ended up in mental hospitals, so why can't it happen to you? There's nothing strong or clever or special about you.

I was shivering; the air on the bus seemed icy. I hadn't known it would be so cold here.

I searched my bag for pills but I hadn't brought them. How I wished I'd something, anything, that might blunt the edges of pain for tonight, be it gin or pills or some grass to smoke. I'd never taken illicit drugs. But what did abstaining from pot and the like matter now that I was living on daily doses of drugs which were probably far more potent than 'soft' drugs like marijuana?

I went to lie on the back seat where there was more room and closed my eyes tightly, willing sleep to come to blot everything out.

Time passed. How long? An hour? Several hours?

As if awaking from a trance, I sat up with a jolt. What was I doing here? I had to go home.

I was outside roaming dark, lonely streets in the early hours of the morning, lost in a street lined with derelict buildings. I glanced behind me. A shadow shifted revealing a man in a dark overcoat. I walked faster. A tense, tingling sensation crept through my body. I jerked round. The gap between us had narrowed. I feared coming to a dead-end. I'd had nightmares like this.

I turned a corner, climbed over a wall near a boarded-up warehouse, stumbled in the dark across a yard, squeezed through a fence and ran along deserted moonlit streets. Exhausted and with a stabbing pain in my side, I could go no further. I stopped near a block of empty houses awaiting demolition and leant, panting, against a wall overlooking a paved yard. After resting there, I hurried along and came to the comparative safety of a familiar main road. I was several miles from home but was able to find my way in the steadily increasing light of early morning.

Dad was setting off for work when I arrived home. He showed no surprise on seeing me and I guessed (rightly as I found out later) that my parents had assumed I'd gone to a disco with Jackie or Mandy and then slept at one of their houses, as I often did.

'Don't you and Brian be noisy today,' Dad said. 'Your mum's in bed with a migraine.'

'She's always got a bleedin' headache,' Brian commented.

'I don't wonder, living here,' I said.

I opened the pantry door and began eating a slice of bread,

too hungry to bother buttering it. After a few mouthfuls I saw the green mould and flung it down in disgust.

'Aren't you going to finish it?' Brian asked.

'No, 'cos the bloody bread's green.'

Brian laughed loudly.

'Shut up, you'll wake Mum.'

'How can it be red if it's green, or green if it's red?'

'What?'

'Don't you get it? It's a joke. You called it *bloody* bread. Blood is red but mould is green. What a face, Jean. You've no sense of humour these days.'

I filled my hot-water bottle and went upstairs. Oh, the bliss of hugging something warm. I pulled an old overcoat of Dad's over my dirty, crumpled clothes, slipped off my shoes and crawled into bed. Outside my room Brian continued his silly talk.

'Hey, Jean, you said the bloody bread was green, didn't you? Blood is red, not green. Don't you know that? So was the bread red or green? Tell me that, then. You can't, can you?'

He showed no signs of ending this monologue so I got out of bed, opened the door, and said softly, 'Be quiet, Brian. You'll wake Mum and she's not well.'

'No one tells me to be quiet! I'll make as much bleedin' noise as I want,' Brian said loudly.

'Oh, you stupid ass!' I said before climbing back into bed.

'That must mean you want to hear my ass noises,' Brian said. He stomped into my bedroom and leant over my bed going 'Hee-haw! Hee-haw! Hee-haw ...!'

I was shivering and aching all over. The last thing I wanted was Brian around. About five minutes later he was still hee-hawing beside my bed and I made the mistake of saying, 'Shut up, you fuckin' swine!' which promptly caused the hee-haws to turn to oinks.

'Oh, I'm a pig now, am I, Jean? All right then. Oink! Oink! Oink! Oink! Oink!'

When he finally left my room, I lay on my back, feeling hot, silent teardrops escaping from the sides of my eyes and trickling into my ears: tears of self-pity because I felt cold and sick and isolated, so achingly, despairingly miserable. I reached for the bottles on my bedside orange-box and swallowed the handful of pills which would transport me to my temporary haven of oblivion.

LOOKING BACK 3

I WAS VERY CLOSE to my father. Among my earliest memories are those of him lying with his head over the arm of the sofa while I, pretending to be his barber, combed his thick, black hair. We also played hide and seek, and he carried me up to bed on his shoulders.

But his 'bad moods' frightened me. Sometimes he'd wake me in the middle of the night, claiming my bed. I'd go into the 'big bed' but Mum would say, 'If yer dad's sleeping in your bed, I'm sleeping downstairs.' I could never understand why she preferred the small, lumpy sofa to sleeping with me. And why did Mum and Dad keep hurting each other? School in the morning. Tired at my desk. Questions unanswered.

I didn't see why God couldn't step in and sort out the troubles at home. But even back then, as early as the age of ten, the first big doubt was already tugging at my sleeve. How could I know for certain that God, unlike Santa Claus, really did exist? One afternoon, alone in the living room, I decided to settle the matter by a little experiment. After all, if angels appeared before mere mortals in biblical days, then why not now?

'Listen, God, I'm going to count up to three,' I told Him, 'and on the count of three, let an angel come into this room, then I'll never doubt again. OK?'

I took a deep breath and counted. One. Two. Three.

Exactly on the count of three the door opened. Startled, I almost screamed in fright. In came my father who tossed a white paper bag into my lap. 'A little present for you,' he said. I opened it with trembling fingers. Inside the bag was an angel.

The kind that is put on Christmas trees and shines in the dark.

Inspired by Captain Costello of the David and Goliath sketch, I wanted to star in our Sunday school plays. Despite my shyness I could speak out loudly and clearly when acting. Mum and Dad were at the adult meeting to watch me when I led a group to follow the Bethlehem Star in our nativity play. My Sunday school teacher decided I would look more the part if I had a long, black pigtail. She pulled a black, nylon stocking on my head, the 'leg part' dangling down my back. When I made my entrance someone at the back of the hall sniggered and then loud laughter erupted throughout the congregation. Bravely, I launched into my eloquent speech, which I had practised every day to reach perfection. After a few sentences I was struggling not to laugh. Unfortunately, people remained more interested in the stocking on my head than the Star in the East.

'Dad, did I do all right?' I asked him afterwards.

'You were wonderful,' he said, hugging me. He was in a good mood that day.

Sometimes Dad's moods were something to do with Mum and Norman Cockroft, a bread-delivery man, who was supposedly a friend of Dad's. Mr Cockroft started coming to our house a lot when Dad was doing the late bus-conducting shift.

I ran from school to arrive home early one day, eager to tell Mum I'd got a gold star for coming top of the ten-year-olds in an English test. On hearing her in the bedroom I slung my gabardine over a chair-back and rushed upstairs. Mr Cockroft's head was peeping round the bedroom door, and he wouldn't let me in. I pushed at the door and caught a glimpse of Mum. She was half-undressed!

Mum giggled in a strange, silly sort of way, while he shouted at me to go away.

'I'll see to her,' Mum said. She appeared in her dressing-gown, led me downstairs and locked me outside after pushing my tortoise into my hand, telling me to feed him on the grass. Sitting among the weeds in our back garden, I tickled Timmy's chin with a clover leaf while gazing at the bedroom window and puzzling over the funny ways of grown-ups.

'You'll catch your death of cold sitting there with no coat on,' Mrs Jessop called over the fence.

'I'm not cold,' I said, wondering why I was lying.

I waited for Mrs Jessop to go, then picked up an apple core and threw it at the bedroom window several times. Mr Cockroft opened the window and the rotten apple core smacked him in the face. I hadn't meant that to happen, but couldn't help giggling.

'Bugger off, yer cheeky kid!'

'Norman! Don't swear at her,' I heard Mum say.

Mum's pale, thin face appeared at the window in place of Mr Cockroft's red, fat face. 'Jean, love, will you fetch me some nylon stockings from Turner's in Bass Street?'

'Can't I have me tea first? I'm hungry.'

'Well, I'll tell you what. Go fetch some ginger biscuits so you can have some with your tea.'

'I don't want any biscuits. How much longer will you be?'

She sighed, shut the window and drew the curtains. I looked down enviously at Timmy's safe, warm shell as I pinched my cold arms and legs, wiped my nose on my sleeve and resigned myself to waiting.

I never mentioned this to Dad because, although I didn't really understand what was going on, I knew it was one of the things that would put him in a bad mood.

'Has he been round again?' Dad said crossly to Mum, eyeing the packets of freshly baked bread rolls on the kitchen table. 'I've told him to only come when I'm in. The neighbours'll be talking.'

'He only came to bring us some bread,' Mum said.

That night, with the covers of the 'big bed' pulled up over my head, I gazed on the luminous angel in my hand until I fell asleep.

CHAPTER TEN

A NEW DECADE, THE seventies, had begun, and soon the long teen years would be over. But here was I, nearing my twentieth birthday, loaded with drugs, robotised, and still seeing Dr Prior.

'I saw you in Smith's on Saturday by the magazine racks,' Dr Prior said, beaming pleasantly, 'and you seemed all right.'

He sounded surprised that I 'seemed all right'. I wondered how else he thought I might behave when out with a friend.

'Are you shy with me when you come here?' he asked.

'Yes,' I said, staring at the desk. Perhaps he'd noticed my body language was 'normal' with Mandy and at last realised my signs of 'nerves' with him were largely due to shyness. That's what I'd tried to tell him several times before.

'Who were you with?'

'Oh, that was Mandy, a friend I've known since school.'

'Do you ever go out with friends in the evenings?' he asked.

'Yes, often,' I replied. 'We go to pubs, dances, places like that.'

'You do? That's wonderful.'

I couldn't see what was wonderful about it, or why he was suddenly interested in something I'd always been doing.

'I can't enjoy myself when I'm tired all the time and, anyway, it all seems wrong somehow.'

'But why is it wrong? Do you think God will punish you for enjoying yourself?'

'No, it's not that,' I said. 'And, anyway, I didn't mean "wrong" in a moral sense.' I stopped, feeling confused. 'At least I don't think I did,' I added, wondering if I did feel guilty about the kind of life I was living.

'Well, what *did* you mean?'

'I meant it all seems so empty and futile and meaningless.'

'I see,' he said, writing something on the papers he always kept in front of him on his desk. It seemed they'd got quite a file on me now. 'So you're still very depressed, Jean, aren't you?'

'Yes, I am,' I agreed.

'I want you to have some more ECT.'

'No!'

'You don't need to go back into hospital for it. You can have it as an outpatient,' he pointed out.

'I don't want any more ECT,' I said firmly. This was one of the few things in life about which I was certain.

'At least consider it,' he said, sounding exasperated. 'I've taken a special interest in your case and discussed it with colleagues. They all think we should try more ECT.'

'Do they really?' I said, feeling uneasy that doctors who didn't know me, had never even seen me, should form opinions like that based on no real knowledge of me or my circumstances.

'Yes, they do,' he said. 'So let's try it, shall we?'

I shook my head vigorously. 'I don't want any more ECT.'

Dr Prior looked tired. He lit a cigarette and began doodling a circular design on his notepad, while I shuffled my feet in the awkward silence.

'I think I'll try adding a new drug.' He wrote something down, then gave me the prescription. 'Who gives you your pills?'

'I don't know what you mean.'

'Well, does your mother keep them and allocate each dose to you when it's due?'

'Oh no, I just take them myself.'

'You have access to the whole lot?'

I nodded. It would never have occurred to my parents to limit my access to the drugs or supervise my dosage. Dr Prior obviously hadn't a clue about my home life despite his 'special

121

interest' in my 'case'.

My brother became the proud owner of a second-hand Mini. He surprised us by showing an aptitude for driving, passing his test the first time. Despite his continuing frequent antagonism towards me, he did sometimes help me out by giving me lifts. One day we were driving down a busy main road when a cat dashed out and was hit by a passing car. I watched, horrified, as other cars missed by fractions the tortoiseshell form in the middle of the road.

Brian jerked to a stop by the kerb. The poor animal tried to stand, wobbled, and slumped back down again. Traffic was notoriously heavy and fast on this stretch of road. It wasn't a place where pedestrians would be likely to risk trying to cross.

'We'll have to find a phone box,' I said.

Brian got out of the car, his eyes on the cat. He stepped into the road.

'Don't! It's too dangerous!' I yelled from the window.

He ignored my cries of alarm. To him there was no choice. 'We can't leave it there,' he said.

Brian dodged the traffic and gently picked up the cat. Horns blasted, cars missed them by inches. I held my breath as he made his way back to the car. Very gently he put the wounded cat on the back seat, covering it with his jacket. I'd never seen such caring concern on his face, such gentle compassion in his eyes.

Back at the wheel, he kept looking over his shoulder at the distressed animal. 'Oh, God, I hope the vet's still open,' he said.

About fifteen minutes later we were pulling up outside the PDSA. Brian lifted the cat carefully, speaking to it in gentle soothing tones each time it whimpered.

'Leave it with me,' the vet said, placing a hand on Brian's shoulder. 'You've done all you can.'

Back in the car, Brian turned on the ignition with a shaky hand.

'Wait a few minutes. Don't start driving just yet,' I urged

him.

'Why not? I'm all right,' he said. But tears had filled his eyes.

'It'll be OK with the vet. It won't be suffering now,' I said.

We resumed our journey, for the most part in silence. I was intrigued by this other Brian, this person with a kind, gentle side to his nature.

'The poor thing,' he said. 'The poor thing.'

One afternoon the world blurred and the room started spinning. I lay on my bed feeling sick, my heart thumping wildly. Pink and yellow lights flashed before my eyes. I rolled on to my stomach and pressed my face, with eyes shut tight, into my pillow. And then came a screeching siren, a shrill whistling sound piercing my brain. I clamped my hands over my ears. It wouldn't stop. My body was shaking. Surging fears of death or madness overwhelmed me. And then all went black.

When I opened my eyes the noise and feelings had subsided, leaving me soaking in perspiration and hardly daring to move. A fit? Gingerly, I crawled off my bed and was relieved to find that, apart from feeling weak, I seemed OK now, but I decided to visit my GP, Dr Russo, that evening.

'It was probably a physical reaction against drugs which are too strong for you,' Dr Russo explained. 'Hardly surprising really. You're on a mixture of potent drugs.'

'Dr Prior added a new one recently. Do you think it's that?'

'Probably. You'd better discontinue it at once.' He leant back in his chair and looked at me. 'How are you feeling?'

'I'm still depressed and Dr Prior wants me to have more ECT,' I said flatly. 'But I don't want it.'

'Well, why not, if that's what the psychiatrist advises?'

'How would you like your brain to be wired up to electricity?' I asked.

Dr Russo smiled. 'Oh, it's not done so primitively,' he said. 'You don't feel anything under the anaesthetic, do you?'

'No, but it's unpleasant when the anaesthetic starts taking effect and then later you wake up feeling terrible. I'm scared

123

it's damaged my brain. I met this lad, James, who apparently I dated a few times a bit back, and he looked at me as if I was some kind of nut because I couldn't even remember going out with him.'

Dr Russo threw back his head and laughed. 'Well, you should go out with him again and enjoy it this time round,' he said.

'It's frightening not to be able to remember things.'

'Are you still seeing that pastor?' Dr Russo asked, changing the subject.

'He visits me occasionally.'

'He can't give you *his* faith.'

'I know.'

'All you need is a nice boyfriend. Once you get married and have children, you'll be all right.'

'I don't want a boyfriend, I don't want to get married and I don't want babies,' I said, feeling irritated at his implication that marriage and babies were all a female could ever want or need.

Dr Russo stroked his chin. 'You know what your parents' marriage has been like and it's put you off. But you shouldn't judge all marriages by theirs.'

'Of course I shouldn't, and I don't,' I said. 'But I want something more in life than marriage and babies.'

'And what is it that you want?'

'I don't know.'

Mike Conway was a mate of one of Jackie's old boyfriends. Tall, dark-haired, not bad-looking, talkative, too self-confident (I was wrong about the latter) were my first impressions of him. I was a jeans-and-casual-tops type, whereas he wore smart suits (and even waistcoats), but I warmed to his friendliness and we started dating regularly.

I was a blank girl, my 'self' eroded by daily cocktails of drugs more deadly than I realised. But my explanation to Mike that I was 'on Valium' seemed to satisfy him, perhaps because repeat prescriptions for tranquillisers weren't unusual at that time. Valium was in fashion. I didn't tell Mike I was a psychiatric patient. No, of course not. Best to keep that hidden away like a guilty secret. Neither did I speak of my soul-sick despair, which I tried to conceal behind jokes and laughter during our long, boozy nights at pubs and nightclubs.

I admitted to Mike that I was unemployed 'at present' but didn't say how long the 'at present' had gone on for. Every Thursday morning I dragged myself out of bed to go to the Employment Exchange to 'sign on', and occasionally they'd send me upstairs to see the Disablement Resettlement Officer, a sweet, grey-haired lady who specialised in finding jobs for the disabled. The conversation with her usually went along the same lines. 'Ah, yes, we do have a vacancy for a clerical post. Oh, but wait a minute. It says the work is high pressure. I think perhaps it would be too stressful for you, wouldn't it?'

'I don't know. I don't want a boring job.'

'No, of course you don't, but let's be realistic, shall we? You've been ill for a long time and you're on medication. We want a nice little job you can manage, don't we?'

It had been Dr Prior's idea that I registered as a disabled person. It would, he said, help me get a job because the law required employers to take on a certain percentage of disabled people. So now I was the owner of a green card to show to prospective employers as proof of a registered disability. I still couldn't take it all in. Was that really my name on this card? Who am I now? A disabled person? And mentally disabled too; a highly stigmatised form of disability. Would I always be separate, different from the world of 'normal' people who didn't think or feel like me and didn't carry a green card?

In April 1970, a year after my discharge from Thornville Ward, I got a job as a stock records clerk at Dobson's, a local engineering firm. I worked alone in a small basement office with damp, peeling walls. There was a constant draught from under the door and the one-bar electric fire at my feet did little more than help warm my toes. My job consisted of simple arithmetic to keep stock-record cards up to date, invoice typing and filing. It was dreadfully boring, but I was determined to

125

prove that, mentally disabled or not, I could hold down a job.

The two warehouse lads, Jeff and Jim, who were also the tea boys, told me tales of the rats and mice they'd seen around the place. Jeff took me to see the tea room one day. It was disgustingly dirty.

'Jim and me have great fun making the drinks,' he said. 'If you knew half the things we get up to. One day we found a dead mouse, still warm, on the floor there and you'll never guess what we did with it.' He was doubled up laughing. 'We dipped it into the gaffer's coffee. Isn't that funny?'

My stomach turned cartwheels at the thought of a mouse that was probably disease-ridden and crawling with lice being dipped into someone's coffee.

'It's horrible!' I said, aghast.

Trying to work, even doing this simple job, while so drowsy with drugs was a big problem. I tried taking my lunchtime dose at teatime and my teatime dose at supper-time, but still often felt too tired to work. Sometimes I would lock myself in the large toilet-cum-washroom, give part of the lino a quick dust with a paper towel, then allow myself the luxury of lying down on the floor and dozing off for ten to fifteen minutes. This must seem ludicrous to most people, but anyone who has experienced the utter fatigue which drugs can induce will understand how tempting it was to lie down on the cold, hard floor and allow heavy, drooping eyelids to close, if only for a short while.

Sometimes I couldn't – simply couldn't – force myself to get back to my desk until I'd splashed my face in icy-cold water and swallowed several caffeine pills, which I found I could obtain from any chemist without a prescription. Caffeine pills were surely no more harmful than drinking plenty of strong coffee, which I'd long been having to do to keep awake.

When I next saw Dr Prior he asked me what my parents thought about my problems. I shrugged my shoulders and fiddled with my hair. 'Dunno. They've enough problems of their own.'

'What kind of problems?'

'Well, marital for instance. Mum's having an affair. They've both had affairs in the past.'

'Really? What makes you think that?'

'Dad told me himself about his. Mum isn't trying to hide this affair she's having now.'

'And she's had others in the past?'

'Maybe only one other. I remember when I was about ten, I found Mum in the bedroom with Dad's friend. She locked me out until ... until they'd finished.'

'Why didn't you tell me this before?' he asked, stubbing his cigarette out with more force than necessary.

'I didn't think it was relevant.'

'But this could have a *traumatic* effect on a child's mind!' he said, waving his hand dramatically. 'A most *traumatic* effect! Oh, you should have told me before, you silly girl.'

Without even writing down what he thought was so important, Dr Prior swiftly packed the papers on his desk into his briefcase, sighed, stood up abruptly and left the room. I sat there alone for a while before going to the reception desk, wondering if the interview was actually over.

The thin-faced receptionist with plum-coloured fingernails flicked through the pages of the appointments diary. 'You'll be seeing a new female doctor, Dr Armstrong, next time,' she informed me. 'That will be in three months. Dr Prior will have moved on to another hospital by then.'

A strange farewell ...

On the way home I kept thinking of Dr Prior's words. 'A most traumatic effect!' It seemed there were many things in my past he might have said the same about. So many traumatic effects. So much damage done to an innocent child. What hope was there for me? Who knew what dangerous demons of the past were lurking deep inside me ready to break out one day? Hurt and anger surged through me. Yes, of course it must have had a traumatic effect on poor little ten-year-old me.

When I got home I was bad-tempered with Mum and continued to brood about it in a disco that night. But gradually this perspective shifted and I began to wonder if I'd been more disturbed by Dr Prior's remarks about the incident than by the incident itself.

Mandy's sixteen-year-old sister, Donna, started with 'psychiatric problems' and was admitted to Dolby Grange, a new mental hospital with a catchment area for people from the south side of the city.

'I don't know what's happening to our Donna,' Mandy told me sadly. 'She imagines she can see and hear things and thinks people are plotting against her. She's on a drug called Largactil and they're going to try ECT.'

Several weeks later, when Donna was spending weekends at home, I was invited for tea at Mandy's.

'I'd better warn you that Donna might not recognise you,' Mandy said, her eyes glistening with tears. 'She's a schizophrenic. That's what her psychiatrist told me mum and dad. He said schizophrenia is an extremely serious mental illness but that it can often be controlled, to a large extent, by drugs. He thinks she'll have to keep taking drugs for the rest of her life.'

'The rest of her life?'

'Yes. To prevent relapses. He said if she stops taking the drugs she'll have to go back into hospital.'

Donna was sitting pale and still, staring at the TV screen, when I entered the room.

'Donna, say hello to Jean,' Mandy's mother said, but Donna remained motionless as a statue. 'Jean knows exactly how you feel. She's been through a nervous breakdown herself, so she'll be able to help you.'

I didn't know how to respond. I wished I could help, but of course I did not know exactly how Donna felt, possessed no magic key that could reach her and had no words of reassurance to offer Donna or her family.

'I'll put the kettle on,' Mandy said, standing up.

An hour later Donna's cup of tea remained on the carpet at

her feet untouched. She still hadn't said a word or altered her stiff, immobile stance. The last time I'd seen her had been about eight weeks ago at a party at her cousin Sarah's house. Watching her gaily mingling with the crowd, I'd envied her because she hadn't seemed shy. Where had that extrovert, vivacious teenager gone?

More time passed. Then the room filled with heart-rending sobs as the stone statue dissolved away into a flood of tears. Thank goodness she hasn't gone so far away that she can't even cry, I thought.

'Don't cry, Donna. I'm right here beside you,' Mandy's mother said, putting her arm round her daughter.

'Don't send me back to that place,' Donna said between sobs. 'Oh, please don't send me back there.'

'But you'll have to go back to the hospital for a while to help you get well. Why are you crying, Donna?'

'I don't know.'

'But you must know. Come on, love, try to tell your mother.'

'Because I'm scared,' said a voice barely audible.

'Don't be silly, love. There's nothing to be scared about.'

I was scared, too. Scared that, like Donna, I'd be fogged up with mind-deadening drugs for the rest of my life. No autonomy. Too tired to live. Isolated and imprisoned in this cotton-wool haze for the rest of my life. No! I couldn't bear this soul-death any longer. So despite Dr Prior's earlier warning about 'slipping back' and despite my promise to him, I knew I *had* to stop taking the pills.

I stopped them all at once. It never occurred to me that perhaps I should do it gradually. This resulted in a rebound from too much sleeping to insomnia. I got through five days at work punctuated by lying in bed thrashing about and staring at the ceiling the whole night long. By the end of the week I felt ready to crawl up the wall and hang like a bat from the rafters.

I stuffed some pills down my throat.

Goddamnit, Dr Prior must be right; I *do* need the drugs, I thought sadly, yet I feel so awful when I take them. There seemed no way out. It was a Catch-22 situation.

LOOKING BACK 4

NEW INTERESTS SUCH AS *pop stars, clothes and hairstyles began to take the place of my old childhood games, I started worrying about pimples instead of Julia beating me at 'dares', and my taste in magazines turned to* Valentine *from* Bunty.

When my family were out, I sang and danced with my friends in our living room to pop music blasting out from a crackly transistor tuned in to Radio Luxembourg. This was shortly before the Beatles leapt to fame. Favourites of mine at the time were Cliff Richard singing 'Do You Wanna Dance?', Susan Maughan's 'Bobby's Girl' and Carole King with 'It Might As Well Rain Until September'.

In bed at night, I rubbed my fingers over my nipples. They stood up like firm, young buds, pleasurable to touch. My friends and I huddled together in the playground discussing our developing breasts and whispering about this mysterious adult thing called Sex. Mr Watson, our Scripture Knowledge teacher, decided to inform us, his class of twelve-year-olds, about the 'facts of life'. Diagrams of a penis before and during erection appeared on the blackboard, causing a few embarrassed giggles. After only one interesting lesson the headmaster put a stop to it. Angry parents were complaining and a great fuss was made, so here endeth our sex education. The nearest we got to this subject in biology lessons was learning about the night life of a frog.

I got dressed for school downstairs in front of the fire, stepping out of my pyjamas and flinging them on a chair. I was late that morning. Julia and Carrie knocked at our door before I was

131

ready. Mum, who was on leave from her mill job, let them in.

'Won't be a sec,' I said, dragging a comb through my tangled hair.

'Hey, look at this!' Mum said, holding out my pyjama bottoms, the crotch of which was covered in blood.

Joking to hide my embarrassment from my friends, I said to Mum, 'Oh God, you'd better get an ambulance, hadn't you?' Behind Mum's back, I grinned and winked at Julia and Carrie. 'Quick Mum! I'm bleeding to death!''

'No, it's nowt to worry about,' Mum said. 'It only means you're growing up. You've started.'

I feigned puzzlement. 'Started what?'

Julia and Carrie looked on and giggled.

'Started having what's called your periods,' she said. 'Blow me! I thought you were far too young to start.'

'I'm nearly a teenager,' I reminded her.

I waddled to school with a bulky makeshift sanitary towel stuffed down my knickers. Mum had made it for me from material cut from an old underskirt, and (in more ways than one) it was bloody uncomfortable. What I was supposed to do with the thing when I went to the toilet, I'd no idea. To make things worse, I kept getting spasms of stomach cramp throughout the day. I didn't like this part of 'growing up'. Not one bit.

Next day was better though. I swallowed an aspirin after my Weetabix, wore my new sanitary belt, and a towel from the packet of Dr White's that Mum had bought me from the corner shop. It seemed now that coping with my periods would be easy-peasy compared with sorting out my new, disturbing thoughts.

I did most of my thinking in bed at night. Lying on my back gazing up at the night sky through the gap between my curtains, I tried to sort out my views on topics such as the colour bar, capital punishment and the existence of God. With friends I still giggled a lot and acted silly, but inside a change was taking place. I was questioning things I had long accepted, especially about God.

The Christmas angel might have settled the issue for me when I was ten, but now, two years later, I could smile at the coincidence and see that it proved nothing. I buried my head in the pillow. 'God, are you really there?' I whispered, and the silence of the room hung heavily in the air.

I stopped going to the Salvation Army when I was nearing thirteen. I wrote in my diary that this was because I needed to learn about other religions and think things over for myself. It could also have had something to do with the less noble reason of preferring to go out with friends.

Sneaking into the cinema by the back door to watch 'X' films became more appealing than going to Sunday school. Not paying is stealing, you're under-age, and this is the Lord's Day *screamed my spoilsport of a conscience while the man with an iron hook instead of a hand climbed from one window ledge to another of a New York skyscraper. I gasped when he almost fell. Would he manage to get through the window to murder that woman? Was I really committing at least three sins at once by being here? He fell, scraping the wall with his hooked hand all the way down to the ground. 'Sorry I'm here, Lord, please forgive me,' I whispered to Jesus. 'Great film, isn't it?' I whispered to Jackie.*

'Armageddon. That word's in the Bible,' I said. 'It's in the Book of Revelation. Means the end of the world.' I was showing off with knowledge gained from years of going to the Sally Army. But Jackie was too preoccupied to be impressed. We were holding a whispered discussion in the school cloakroom. She'd brought a newspaper article to show me titled 'Children of the Bomb' in which our generation was described as being the first to grow up under the shadow of the atom bomb. It said we were 'heading straight towards Armageddon'.

'Look, Jean. It says that never before has our planet been in such danger.' Jackie chewed at her thumb nail. She always did that when thinking hard. 'If the bomb goes off before we get home today, we'll never see our families again.'

It was scary to think we might not reach our front gates on the way home from school. Talking about it made it more real. I couldn't imagine how dying would feel. I'd never died before. Or if I had I couldn't remember.

'Do you think we've lived before?' I asked Jackie, who was still biting her nail. 'I've been reading a library book about reincarnation. Some people believe that when we die we come back to earth again as a baby.'

'Well, if we do keep coming back, we won't this time, will we? I mean there'll be no earth to come back to if it's a nuclear war.'

I thought about it. A whole lot of souls lined up and squashed together like in the Saturday matinee cinema queue. All waiting to be sent back to earth. Only there was no earth left to come back to. I didn't know if that was funny or sad. But the thought of nuclear war wasn't funny. 'Oh, Jackie. Don't.'

The more we talked about it that day among the coats hanging lifeless on their pegs, the more it bothered us. Funny how being nearly thirteen and starting your periods makes you bother about things.

CASE NO. 10826

Had a normal childhood untill [sic] she was about 13. She had friends and could mix very well. Since she changed school at 13 she became acutely disturbed by the feeling that she is not welcomed by the girls at the other school which she changed to at 13. She remained isolated and did not mix at all well. Did not like games and sports.

Dr Prior

CHAPTER ELEVEN

'WHAT ARE YOU THINKING about?' Mandy asked as we trudged around town on a shopping expedition one cold Saturday.

'Oh, just an old joke I once heard,' I replied with a cynical smile. 'The treatment was successful but the patient died.'

'I knew you weren't listening to me,' Mandy said. 'I was saying you don't look at all well.'

'I'm OK,' I said, shivering in a chilly breeze.

'But you're *not* OK. You look like death warmed up.'

'Death warmed up?' I laughed. 'Well, that'd be an improvement. I'm not even warmed up.'

A snowstorm started. I giggled as an Asian man walked past us with a newspaper pulled down firmly over the top of his head and a facial expression that said exactly what he thought of English winters.

'Well, I'm glad you haven't lost your sense of humour,' Mandy said, brightening up. 'C'mon, Jean, let's go for dinner.'

'Do you think my illness might be similar to Donna's?' I asked Mandy as we sat in a Wimpy Bar indulging in our latest craze: cheeseburgers. Mandy's sister had been discharged from hospital looking as I had: fat and sleepy. Although Donna's symptoms were different, her treatment – ECT and the drugs such as Melleril and Largactil – was the same.

'No, of course not,' Mandy replied promptly. 'Donna's got schizophrenia, not depression. You do both sometimes look kinda distant, but I always get a sensible answer when I talk to you. With Donna it's completely different. She thinks foreigners are taking over the country.'

'Sounds like the way me dad and our Brian talk,' I said.

'But Donna's too ... too intense about it. And, anyway, it's not only that. Sometimes she talks to people who aren't there. Oh, Jean, you don't know the half of it. Schizophrenia is the most terrible illness.'

I nodded sympathetically, wishing I could think of something helpful to say. How awful it must be for Donna and her family.

But why, I wondered, with Donna's illness obviously so different from mine, was our treatment the same?

I looked forward to seeing my new psychiatrist, Dr Armstrong, because a different person would have a fresh outlook. Or so I thought. A bespectacled, middle-aged woman, with light-brown curly hair framing a pink, roundish face, was seated behind the desk in place of Dr Prior. She nodded for me to sit down, then continued to read my notes.

'I think I'll try changing your medication,' she announced finally.

I wondered if she'd been one of Dr Prior's colleagues who, without even seeing me, thought I should have more ECT. She obviously viewed me as already classified, and needing medication, before even bothering to look at or listen to me.

'You've been on the same tablets for a long time and they don't seem to be doing any good, do they?' she muttered, half to me half to herself, unaware of my disappointment in her. 'We'll try changing your Melleril to chlorpromazine.'

'Will the new pills make me less drowsy and depressed?' I asked, a faint hope rising in me. I wasn't aware then that chlorpromazine was another name for Largactil, a drug I'd been on before the Melleril, which had made me feel equally awful.

'Well, all these kind of drugs have a sedative effect, but I can include something for the depression.' She was still leafing through the pages in front of her. 'Actually, you've never been on antidepressants.'

'Really? What kind of drugs have I been taking?' I asked.

'Oh, various kinds to reduce anxiety and help you sleep.'

'But I can barely keep awake!' I pointed out.

'I think you need an antidepressant as well. I'll try amitriptyline.'

The drugs sorted out to her satisfaction, she asked me to explain my confusion about religion. I was bored of it myself by now and had long ago stopped thinking a psychiatrist might understand, but I trotted out the old story.

'Hell doesn't exist. The Bible isn't meant to be taken literally: it's full of metaphors,' she said, shaking her head. 'Heaven doesn't exist either. The world's moved on from fairy tales to science.' She sighed. 'But really, love, you ought to have had more sense than to try to believe things like that in the first place, don't you think?'

'Perhaps so,' I replied sadly.

I left, feeling disappointed with Dr Armstrong's preconceived ideas about me and her drugs-orientated approach, and was soon to find that my 'new' drugs, including the red amitriptyline pills, would do nothing to make me feel less drowsy and depressed. If anything, I felt even worse.

Someone must have dipped all the clocks in treacle to slow down time. The hours between starting work at half-past eight and finishing at half-past five seemed to last for ever. It was only half-past two. A pile of stock-record cards littered my desk ready for me to write a few figures into a column on each card. I saw myself doing the same repetitive, unfulfilling tasks day after day, year after year. You ought to be grateful you've got a job; any sort of life is better than being in a mental institution. Yes, I know, but I can't stand it, I can't stand it. Yes, you can, you've got to. No, I simply can't bear another three boring hours here. You must. But I can't, I can't …

Then, impulsively grabbing my bag and coat, I fled from the office and went home.

I was thankful to find no one was in, and lay on my bed staring at the ceiling. For six months I had clung to a job I hated as if it was my last hope of something akin to a normal life. I couldn't have tried harder but I had failed. So what now?

Pastor West called to see me one evening about three months after I'd left my job. I hadn't seen him for some time and soon he and his family would be moving to Scotland.

'I've walked out of my job,' I told him. 'I can't work when I'm so drugged but the psychiatrist says I must keep taking my tablets.'

'You're still on drugs and seeing a psychiatrist?' he asked, sounding surprised. 'Do you think that's helping you?'

'Psychiatry only seems to have made me worse.'

I remembered sitting in the park one crisp, autumn day on my way to that first appointment with a psychiatrist. I wished I could go back in some kind of time warp and find myself, aged eighteen, still sitting there beside the pond that had not yet frozen over. 'Don't go. Don't get involved with psychiatry,' the me with hindsight would warn the old, naïve trusting me. 'It's dangerous.'

'Jean, why don't you stop seeing the psychiatrist?' Pastor West asked, breaking my daydream.

'What? Stop seeing a psychiatrist altogether?' It seems I had forgotten that this option was open to me. I stared at Pastor West as if he'd suggested I fly to the moon. Didn't he realise how ill I was, how awful I felt?

'Yes, why not? You've said yourself that psychiatry only seems to be making you worse, and I'm inclined to agree with you.'

'But I've proved that I'm too sick to hold down even a simple job, haven't I? I can't blame the drugs for everything. I've always been bored with my jobs. Other people have to do boring work and they manage it.'

'Perhaps you've been doing the wrong jobs. Have you ever thought of being a nurse?'

'Fat chance when the only experience I've had of hospitals is as a mental patient.'

'Well, working as an auxiliary would be a start. I'd be happy to give you a reference. Think about it.'

About a week later I received a letter from Pastor West saying he'd spoken to the Matron at a local general hospital and she was willing to interview me. If he didn't hear from me by Tuesday, he'd assume I wanted him to cancel it.

When I went for my next appointment with Dr Armstrong I had a letter in my bag ready to post, agreeing to Pastor West's proposal. It was my father's day off work. He said he'd come to the hospital with me and then we could go for tea afterwards at a fish and chip café.

When I told Dr Armstrong about walking out of my job, her face tightened into a frown. 'You know, Jean, I think you really need to come into hospital again for a while.'

'No!' I said, panic rising in me.

'But the rest would do you good.'

Rest? Oh no, I wasn't going to fall for that one again.

'We could try different types, strengths and combinations of drugs more freely in the hospital where we could keep an eye on you and decide how best to treat you.'

I shuddered at these words, remembering my previous stay.

'Actually, I think we might be able to admit you tomorrow because there's room at the moment in a really lovely ward. If we delay, the vacancy might go and that would be a shame because I'm sure a nice rest would do you the world of good.'

Were we talking about the same place? We were talking about a mental institution and she was making it sound like a holiday camp.

'Do think about it, dear,' she said. 'Thornville's a *lovely* ward.' Much emphasis was placed on the word 'lovely'.

I don't believe this, I thought. Isn't there anyone I can trust? But then, she hadn't seen the hospital from the same angle as me, so perhaps she genuinely did not know.

'That's the ward I was in before and I hated it,' I said icily.

She pushed back her glasses, which had slid to the end of her nose, and frowned. 'Well, all right then. But what will you do? What are you going to do about a job, for instance?'

'I'd like to be a nurse. Well, not a nurse, I know I couldn't do that just now but I mean an auxiliary,' I said hesitantly,

140

feeling myself blush.

'Well, that's a nice thought, dear, but I don't think … Now, how can I put it? You want to work in hospital because you've been in hospital and you want to help people get well, don't you? That's lovely. But I think at the moment we should be looking at how we can get *you* well. I'm certain the best thing for you would be to come back into hospital and get yourself nicely rested.'

'No!' I said, horrified. 'I'd get worse.'

'Is that your father I saw with you?'

'Yes, but he doesn't want me to go back into hospital either,' I said anxiously. I was afraid, as I had been when Sister Oldroyd tried to bully me into having further ECT, that a 'mental illness' diagnosis meant my own wishes and views could be overridden.

She drummed on the desk with her pen. 'Actually, I think there might be an alternative to admission seeing as you're so set against it. How would you feel about attending a day hospital? An ambulance would take you there each morning and bring you back home at teatime.'

'Yes, I'd agree to that,' I said weakly, feeling the last remaining ounce of confidence in my ability to do the sort of job Pastor West had suggested draining out of me. I had given the auxiliary job a lot of thought and had wanted to try it, but now I felt embarrassed at having mentioned it to Dr Armstrong. Of course I couldn't work. I was too sick.

'Now, if you'll take a seat in the waiting area, I'll just have a quick word with your father.'

In the café Dad and I ate our fish and chips in silence for a while. He seemed subdued since speaking to Dr Armstrong.

'What did she say about me?'

'She said you're a nice girl but you're a sick girl,' he replied, his voice trembling a little.

'A sick girl. Yeah, I guess that's right,' I said, prodding the haddock on my plate with my fork while I mourned again the loss of my mental health. The thought I sometimes harboured that maybe my distress wasn't really an 'illness' was fading.

After all, three psychiatrists – Dr Sugden, Dr Prior and Dr Armstrong – couldn't all be wrong.

Could they?

The night after Dr Armstrong had suggested the day hospital, I tried to tell Mike the truth. He thought I was still working at Dobson's. In the Old Crown after several barley wines I managed to steer the conversation to psychiatry. There'd been something on TV recently about psychiatry and teenage depression. It seemed a useful starting point.

'No, I didn't see that programme,' Mike said. 'But I know enough about mental illness.'

'You do?'

'My uncle went off his head. Murdered his fiancée.'

'Murdered her?'

'Yeah. About twenty years ago. He was living with us at the time. I came home from school that day and let myself in. Mum sometimes didn't get back from work till a bit later. I opened the living-room door. Blood everywhere. Carpet. Sofa. Even the curtains.'

'Oh, Mike. How awful!' I reached out and squeezed his hand.

'Anyway, they sent him to Broadmoor and operated on his brain. Turned him into a suitably safe cabbage. He's in High Royds now.'

'High Royds?'

'Yes. A strange place. But it's a good job there are such hospitals. They do their best for the poor sick buggers.' He took a few gulps of beer. 'They even put on dances for them. You won't believe this but there's a large ballroom actually inside the hospital.'

'Is there?' I asked blankly. I'd been to one of these dances myself when an in-patient.

'Yes, really,' he said knowledgeably.

Mike went to fetch more drinks. I closed my eyes and saw it all again. People sitting on fold-up chairs around the sides of the hall rocking back and forth, writhing, grimacing, twisting, looking as if their mouths were stuffed full of chewing gum; inmates staggering around to the sound of a band playing 'White Christmas'; the staff joining in. Oh yes, they'd tried: paper hats, streamers, balloons and … Lord, the terrible sadness was almost tangible

Me at eighteen. Newly admitted. Shoved down the rabbit hole into a world like nothing I could have imagined. I had found a vacant chair next to a woman who was jerking and drooling. I sat gulping water from a polystyrene cup, though a side effect of Largactil ensured that my mouth remained distressingly dry. But, hey, I was lucky. Better dry than drooling. Achingly, I'd watched sad-eyed patients in fancy hats doing a Largactil shuffle across the dance floor. Dreaming of a white Christmas? Hardly.

Another memory of that Christmas dance. Me 'waltzing' around the hall with a man with vacant staring eyes. I hadn't wanted to hurt his feelings by refusing to dance. It might have taken him courage to ask. He held me stiffly and moved like a robot. We shuffled around the polished, wooden floor, out of step with the music and, as I looked at those strange, lifeless eyes that were close to my face, I felt as if I was trying to dance with a corpse.

'Uncle Lionel enjoys those hospital dances,' Mike said, putting our drinks down on the table, 'though he can't keep pace with the music. He shuffles around the dance floor like death-in-life.'

'Ooops!' Back in the present with Mike, I fumbled in my handbag for a tissue to mop up some drink I'd just spilt on the table.

'Relatives can go to these dances. I got invited to one and went along for a laugh,' he said.

'For a laugh? Oh yes, of course. I expect it was very funny.' I don't think Mike even noticed the angry sarcasm in my voice. 'What were the patients like?' I asked.

'Some really sad cases. But others seemed perfectly normal on first impression. I asked a girl to dance. Looked about nineteen, quite pretty. Thought she was a nurse in civvies. It turned out she was a patient.' He shook his head and raised his eyebrows at remembering his mistake. 'Amazing. You wouldn't have thought anything was wrong with her.' He paused to take a swig of his beer. 'Except she talked a load of rubbish,' he added with a smile.

'Oh, did she?' I said, feeling disappointed that he hadn't managed to talk to one of the many patients who didn't talk rubbish.

'Well yes, *of course* she talked rubbish,' he said, sounding surprised at my naivety. 'Don't forget she was a mental patient.'

I finished off my drink quickly. It left a bitter taste. Had the girl really talked rubbish or had it just seemed so to Mike because that's what he'd expected of her? I was definitely not going to tell him about me.

On the night before I was due to start at the day hospital, I went to bed late after spending the evening with Mike. I was sitting up in bed sipping Horlicks and thinking about my life as I gazed through the gap in my curtains at the pale moon, a silvery disc suspended for aeons in a vast expanse of dark sky. The future looked bleak. Tomorrow an ambulance would be drawing up outside our house to take me to the day hospital which stood in the grounds of the main hospital.

'I'm a sick girl,' I whispered into my mug of Horlicks, warming my face in the comforting steam. 'A sick girl. What does that mean? Will I ever get well? Have I ever been well?'

LOOKING BACK 5

'LOOK AT THIS,' JULIA said, thrusting a Daily Mirror at me. There were just the two of us in our kitchen. I looked. It was a photograph of a football crowd.

'I've been thinking,' she said, pushing a stray lock of unruly red hair out of her eyes. 'We could pick one person in the crowd, anyone at all. Take her for instance.' She pointed her finger at a young woman's round, smiling face. 'She's a person just like you and me. She thinks and feels and eats and sleeps and laughs and cries and... Everything about herself and her day-to-day living is as ... er ... as big to her as what our own lives are to us. It's her world. Yet to us she's nothing but a face in a crowd, just as we would be to her. And what I've just said could apply to any single one of the billions of people in the whole world.'

'Yes, I know what you mean,' I said excitedly. Off we went into one of those delightful conversations in which we were cresting the same waves.

And then we began thinking about 'time'. We were thirteen. Soon, tomorrow would be today, and today – this very day now – would be yesterday. Years would pass. We would die. More time would pass. One hundred years. Two hundred years. Today would belong to history. Nobody on earth now would be alive then. And nobody could do anything about time. It just went on and on.

The clock on the mantelpiece ticked loudly.

'Look, it isn't half-past six yet,' said Julia, her greenish-grey eyes wide and serious. 'But it soon will be and there's nothing anyone can do to keep hold of this minute.'

145

'But it isn't half-past six right now, this very second,' I said. I realised I was clenching my fists as if in a futile attempt to capture and hold that minute; to hold in abeyance the past and the future, retaining the NOW. That's when we started working ourselves up into a frenzy, gesticulating madly and raving about it being now, right now, this very second now. Never before had now seemed so now-ish.

But even as we were experiencing this heightened awareness of the present, the clock kept ticking, the minute was spiralling beyond our reach. The red second-hand on the clock moving quietly, steadily, reached and passed the number twelve. We leaned our heads back, exhausted at our wrestling match with Time, and laughed at the way our feelings had reached a pitch of intensity as we'd tried – almost literally – to hold infinity in the palm of our hand.

Time wouldn't stop. Of course it wouldn't. And things were about to change. At age thirteen, the pupils in our class had the option of transferring to a new comprehensive school where we could sit for GCE exams. Notes were sent to inform our parents. My mum and dad, with their usual lack of interest in my schooling, said I could please myself. I tingled with excitement. Rossfields was a 'posh' new school. It even had tennis courts and showers. I loved the idea of bringing books home to do homework. My friends, like most of our class, didn't share my enthusiasm and wouldn't be going. I'd be forced into making new friends and this, I told myself, would be good for me. I planned to try very hard to overcome the painfully intense feelings of shyness I experienced with everyone except my five best friends.

On my first day I knotted my maroon and grey striped tie with pride. It matched the grey skirt and maroon cardigan. I'd never worn a school uniform before and I liked the idea. A uniform, I thought, gave a sense of belonging. I picked up the brown leather satchel I'd bought from a jumble sale, and set off with a mixture of anxiety and optimism. A hole in the bottom left corner of my satchel proved just the right size for my ruler to keep dropping through as I hurried along the paths in the cemetery taking a handy short-cut.

There were about thirty pupils per class, a fairly even mix of boys and girls. The school seemed so big and impersonal, though at my previous schools I'd been in classes of forty. I spent my first week at Rossfields trying to find my way round endless staircases and corridors, trying to remember the names of teachers who wore strange black gowns. And, most important to me, trying to find the courage to speak to my new classmates. Standing alone in the playground, I missed my friends so much.

I did manage to make a new friend in my class. Her name was Mandy; a tall, slender girl with large brown eyes and black curly hair. My hand shook as we held a book we were sharing, and conversation was so hampered by my social anxiety, until, very gradually, my shyness with Mandy lessened. Then, just before the results of the end of term exams were given out, we were told the pupil with the highest marks would go up into the A1 class. That was me!

After the holidays I went to join my new classmates in Room 10. The noise I could hear before entering the room told me the teacher was absent. A girl sitting with her feet up on the desk greeted my arrival by shouting: 'We don't want you in this class.' I sat down self-consciously at the nearest vacant desk and was promptly told to 'shift' by a girl who claimed it was her desk.

Later that day I held back my tears as I walked home through the large cemetery. Crippled by shyness, I became the only pupil sitting alone in every lesson at a double desk; in Cookery I worked alone at a table for four.

Our house was dirty, smelly, and untidy, and, I'm afraid, so was I. I can picture myself with my greasy hair, just long enough to hide my mucky neck, straggling over the grubby collar of my crumpled school blouse. My grey socks were meant to be white, and I wore scuffed hole-in-the-sole shoes. At my old school, who cared? There I'd watched kids as scruffy as myself playing at pulling nits out of their hair, lining them up on their desk, and giggling at the popping sound each egg made beneath the pressure of a thumbnail. But no one cracked nits on the spanking new desks here.

When the schoolgirl teasing turned vicious I was ill-equipped to deal with it. My self-confidence in social situations was smaller than a peanut. I was bullied constantly. Without one single friend in my new class, I drifted away on a piece of flotsam and became an outcast.

And I was losing touch with my five best friends. We'd grown up together: played, laughed, cried, quarrelled, fought, hugged, shared secrets for so long. How could it all just end? I read a Charlotte Brontë poem that reminded me of Rainbow Land days, sensed something precious was fading, and wept.

> We wove a web in childhood,
> A web of sunny air;
> We dug a spring in infancy
> Of water pure and fair...

Of course, there was my new friend, Mandy, with whom I spent summer Saturday afternoons sitting by the lake in the park eating crisps and drinking orange juice. But it wasn't the same: none of the imaginative games or the shared intimacies or the giddy fits of giggling, the whoops of sheer joy.

My diary, the red-bound book with a silhouette of a girl with a ponytail on the cover, became my best friend and confidante. 'I hate being in this class,' I wrote. 'I'm so lonely and miserable.' Around the time I was writing this, my new form teacher was writing on my report: 'Jean is coping admirably with her work and has settled down well in her new class.'

CASE NO. 10826

27 January 1971
Dr T Smith
Consultant Psychiatrist
High Royds Hospital

Dear Dr Smith

re: Miss Jean Davison age 20
....

    I should be very grateful if you would consider taking Miss Jean Davison over as a day patient.

    She suffers from chronic schizophrenia and has been working until three months ago. She is not well enough to go back to work but not ill enough to necessitate admission to hospital. Dr Dean has been consulted in this matter and he would be very pleased if you could find your way clear to accepting her as a day patient.

    Yours sincerely

R Armstrong
Medical Assistant

CHAPTER TWELVE

WHEN THE AMBULANCE ARRIVED at our house I noticed the curtains of a bungalow opposite being pulled to one side. Another neighbour kept turning to look while walking past as a nurse opened the rear door for me. Well, let the nosey parkers stare if they've nothing better to do, I thought irritably.

My old wounds smarted as we turned into the familiar driveway and I saw again those thick stone walls, the imposing frontage of the grim institution. But, instead of bearing left to continue up the main drive, we took a sharp turn to the right and jerked to a halt on a gravel path outside a small, whitewashed building that looked like a detached house enclosed in a neat garden.

A smart-suited man of about forty greeted me at the door. He shook my hand warmly, and introduced himself as Mr Jordan, the day hospital charge nurse. He took me into a room where about ten other patients were sitting round a large table. They were drawing or knitting. Bob Dylan's voice floated out from the radio in the corner singing one of my favourite songs: 'Blowin' in the Wind'.

A young woman was humming along to the radio and I noticed that she, like some of the others, looked to have what today would be called 'learning difficulties'. I felt saddened at the thought of what kind of life people like her must have. It was only when she stopped and looked at me that I realised I'd been staring. I felt uncomfortable.

'Hi! My name's Caroline. What's yours?'

'Jean.'

Caroline had a bad squint and the whites of her eyes kept

showing; that's when you could see her eyes at all, for they were hooded with heavy lids. Despite her loud, extrovert manner it seemed she was heavily drugged. A small, turned-up nose looked to have been stuck on to the pale face. Her short, dark-brown hair, which fell over her forehead in a longish fringe, had been given a 'basin' cut. She was wearing a grey skirt with a white blouse, which reminded me of my old school uniform, and white ankle socks.

'How old are you, Jean?' she asked.

'Twenty.'

'Get away with you! You're pulling my leg, aren't you? You look about sixteen. Only sweet sixteen. Guess how old I am?'

Mr Jordan smiled. 'This one will talk you to death,' he said to me, nodding at Caroline. 'She's driving me crazy.'

'Take no notice of him, Jean. He's only jealous 'cos I beat him at dominoes.'

Some good-natured bantering went on between the two of them, then Caroline returned her attention to me.

'I'm twenty-one and I'm a bit backward,' she said. This last bit of information was given in the same matter-of-fact way as the first. 'I live over yonder in the big hospital. I've lived there a long time. But I *have* got a dad. He's a Youth Leader. Not that he cares owt for me or else he wouldn't have put me away, would he? Mr Jordan got me my job here. I come over every day to make the tea and coffee, wash up and keep the place tidy.'

She started humming the tune of the Dylan song again. After a while she stopped and stared at me. 'I'd like us to be friends, Jean,' she said.

'Yes, I'd like that too,' I said, clasping the trembling nicotine-stained hand, which had been thrust across the table at me. Caroline had the kind of loud voice and raucous laughter that could grate on your nerves, but there was something endearing about her. I liked her for her acceptance of me. She was open and friendly.

Among the patients who were drawing, there was a lad of

151

about nineteen with dark, bushy hair and grey eyes that glittered like steel in the sun. He was trying to draw me. I was given paper and a pencil and told to draw Melvyn, the fair-haired young man sitting opposite me in a trance-like state with his eyes half closed. Melvyn had a fixed smile upon his thin lips, which I found later was his permanent expression.

'He's a happy lad is our Melvyn,' said Mr Jordan. 'Never stops smiling.'

This latter point was proven at lunchtime when Melvyn was sick into his plate and he just sat there retaining his Cheshire cat grin while Sue, a pretty, auburn-haired student nurse, groaned as she cleared his plate away. 'Oh not again! If it's not Geoff, it's you, Melvyn.'

'What do you mean if it's not me?' Geoff, the lad who had been drawing me, looked up indignantly from shovelling huge spoonfuls of sponge pudding into his mouth, using his spoon and his thumb in a way which reminded me of my brother.

'Well, you're often sick, Geoff, through being greedy.' She brushed some crumbs from her lilac woollen mini-dress.

'But if I don't eat the food it goes in the bin,' Geoff said, becoming agitated, 'and I don't believe in wasting food. I've been brought up never to waste food. It's a sin to throw food away when people are starving.'

'Oh, here we go again,' Sue said, smiling.

None of the day hospital staff wore a uniform, and the patients addressed Sue and the other student nurse, Ray, by their first names. This did help to create a better atmosphere than over on the wards but, even so, I couldn't help wondering what I was doing in such a place. What would Mike think if he could see me now?

After lunch and pills we sat in the lounge and most of the patients leant their heads back in the easy chairs and slept. Geoff came and sat in a chair opposite me, studied my face carefully, and continued his drawing. Every now and then he tore up his sheet of paper, strode round the room muttering, banged his fist down heavily on the coffee table (much to the annoyance of the sleeping patients), then started trying to draw me again. During the next hour or so, whenever I glanced across at Geoff I found him studying my face for his sketch. I was relieved when Mr Jordan sent many of the patients, including Geoff, over to the OT department in the main hospital. He told me to stay at the day hospital for today and play draughts with Elsie.

Elsie was an elderly patient, a frail, thin woman who frequently rocked back and forth, and her jaws were constantly engaged in a chewing motion. The draughtboard had been assembled on a small coffee table when Mr Jordan called me over.

'Jean will play draughts with you,' he told Elsie, who looked up and gave me a gummy smile. 'Do you know how to play draughts, Jean?' I nodded. 'Good. I'll leave you to it then,' he said, and left the room.

Elsie had already moved a black draught so I moved a white one but then Elsie also moved a white one.

'Are you black or white?' I asked.

'Oh, I'm sorry,' she said, moving another white one before also moving a black one.

At first I tried to keep the game in some sort of order and teach her to play, but she was too confused. Finding it impossible to get her to understand, I started letting her move whatever and wherever she wanted when it was her turn. Sometimes she thought she'd won, sometimes she thought I'd won. The rules had been turned upside down, abandoned, and, as game after game proceeded in the same haphazard way, I began to feel like Alice in *Alice in Wonderland*. The more fed-up I was getting, the more Elsie seemed to be enjoying herself. Her sad, wrinkled face became animated, she chuckled merrily each time she 'won' and, with the excited enthusiasm of a child, she kept setting the pieces up for another 'game'. About an hour and several games later I'd had more than enough.

'Let's have a rest now,' I suggested, as yet another game came to an end, but Elsie was happily rearranging the pieces.

'This time you can be black and I'll be white,' she said.

I stared at the draughtboard with aching eyes. When I didn't move, Elsie looked at me expectantly.

'Oh, I do like playing with you,' she said. 'I haven't enjoyed myself so much for ages. Go on, Jean. I think it's your turn to move first this time, isn't it?'

Of course I hadn't the heart to refuse.

I was eventually rescued by Caroline's appearance with the tea trolley. After tea break Sue said we'd got time for a few group games before the ambulances came. The patients who had been to the OT department returned and we played a game where Sue asked each of us a question. If we got the answer wrong we had to do a 'forfeit' decided on by Sue. When my turn came to do a 'forfeit' Sue told me to go outside and shout 'Hot peas!' six times. There was nobody nearby in the hospital grounds, thank goodness, but I still felt stupid and stood hesitating on the gravel path by the door.

'Hot peas,' I said self-consciously; it came out in a soft, hoarse voice.

'I said shout it, not whisper it,' Sue reminded me.

'Oh well, it's only a bit of fun,' I told myself, trying to enter into the spirit of the game.

'HOT PEAS! HOT PEAS! HOT PEAS …!'

Everyone laughed. But then the game took a darker turn.

We went back inside and Betsy, a plump, reticent patient, was told to stand in the middle of the floor and jump up and down, turning round, while repeating the words 'I am silly!' She smiled coyly, turned crimson, and looked down at the carpet.

'Come on Betsy. Start now,' Sue urged her.

Poor Betsy began jumping and turning, obviously feeling embarrassed. 'I am silly,' she mumbled.

'No, you've got to keep on saying it until I tell you to stop,' Sue said, giggling. Betsy, looking terribly uncomfortable, paused to catch her breath, then she started jumping round again. 'I am silly! I am silly! I am silly! I am silly …!'

This 'therapy' was interrupted when Mr Jordan came into the room. 'Jean, your ambulance has arrived. Sit down, Elsie, it's not yours. Now, is there anyone else for Bradford? No, it

154

looks like there's only you today, Jean. See you tomorrow.'

The ambulance driver, a balding man with a paunch, winked at me as I climbed inside the rear door. When we rounded the bend in the drive he pulled up, opened the door and beckoned to me. 'Come and sit up front with me, luv,' he said.

He helped me up on to the seat beside him, and resumed driving.

'No point sitting in the back on your own, is there? It's nice to have some company, especially when it's a pretty girl like you.'

His eyes wandered briefly from the road to my knees and I knew I should have stayed in the back. He chatted in a pseudo-friendly manner, swiftly bringing the conversation round to sex.

'Attitudes towards sex have changed, haven't they?' he said. 'When I was young, lasses of your age were mostly virgins but nowadays it's ... well, that's not the fashion today, is it? I bet you've had lots of lovers, haven't you?'

Of course I should have told him to mind his own business and insisted on riding in the back. But I was much too passive in those days. I let him prattle on, wondering if this was his usual 'patter' for any young woman or whether he was trying to take advantage of a mental patient.

'A lot of the lasses I've carried to and from that place are bonkers and sex mad.'

'Are you sure it's them and not you?' I asked coolly.

'Aw, come on luv, don't be offended. I know you aren't like that, but you wouldn't believe what some of them are like. I've lived a lot in my time but some of them can even make *me* blush! I'd a young girl in here a bit since, only about sixteen she was, and she'd had it more times than I've had hot dinners. She kept going on about the size of the penises she'd seen. She said, "You should've seen the cock I saw last night. It was a whopper! I've seen some big 'uns before but, blimey, nowt like this! People tell me I've got a big mouth but I had a job on getting it in that, never mind anywhere else!" Yep, you

155

should've heard her and she couldn't have been a day over sixteen.'

He began to laugh loudly and I gripped the sides of my seat as the ambulance swerved.

'A whopper!' he said, between bursts of foolish laughter. 'Can you imagine it? A whopper!'

The whole world's gone mad, I thought, as his senseless laughter continued. And I've got to learn to live in this sick, crazy world.

LOOKING BACK 6

'YOUR DAD TRIED TO strangle me.'

Mum was sitting on the garden wall, crying, in the middle of the night. I found her there after Dad jerked me from sleep by dragging me out of bed. He barricaded himself in my bedroom, with furniture up against the door.

'Strangle you? Oh, don't be so dramatic.'

'It's true. And that's your father who you think is so wonderful!'

I stood shivering on the doorstep in my pink, baby-doll pyjamas. 'It's cold and dark out here. Come inside, Mum.'

'Not yet.'

I hesitated, then stumbled towards her, wincing as I stepped from cool, damp grass on to sharp pieces of grit. I heaved myself up to sit on the wall beside her, my bare feet dangling above the gravel path. Slipping my arm around her shoulders I let her sob against my chest. But I didn't believe what she'd just told me. I couldn't.

Over the next few days my bedroom remained barricaded. I could hear Dad crying inside. My parents were cracking up. Whom could I talk to? There had never been any other significant adults in my life. No family gatherings, no kisses and cuddles from grandparents, aunts, uncles. As a child I'd been taken to visit my grandparents but remembered no affection from them. They were dead now except for my mother's father, an alcoholic.

So whom could I talk to? Certainly not Brian, who tapped on milk bottles and jingled coins. Who could help my parents? I stared at the living room wall where a watery boiled egg Dad had thrown had splattered down the wallpaper and Mum's attempt to wipe it off had made it worse. 'It has to be me,' I whispered. 'There is only me.'

I went upstairs and listened, nervously, outside the barricaded door. I knocked lightly. No reply. 'It's me, Dad,' I called.

'Go away,' came an anguished voice from inside.

'OK, but I'll come back later. I want to talk to you.'

My aim was to be gently persistent. This approach worked for I was subsequently admitted several times over the next few days. I sat on the bed next to him and held him in my arms while he broke down and cried. His pain became my pain. At first we didn't say much: we just hugged. I was fourteen and still innocently unaware that such physical and emotional closeness as ours could be unhealthy.

'I feel worthless and guilty, and ...' his voice trembled, '... and scared, Jean. Really scared.'

'Scared?'

'Yes. Of losing control. Hitting your mum or summat.'

'But you wouldn't really harm her, would you?' I asked anxiously.

He sobbed while I held him tight.

'I'm no good. Did you know I was a thief? One day in my teens I cycled to a church meeting on a stolen bike with a jar of stolen meat paste in my pocket. Something happened to me in that meeting, Jean. I felt the presence of God; it's hard to explain. I repented in tears and became a Christian.' He paused. The room was silent except for our breathing. 'It was good,' he continued, 'for a long time.' He sighed.

I was waiting for the 'but'. I knew there'd be a 'but'.

'But then I got in with a bad crowd and started sleeping around and stealing again. I've been in prison for house-breaking. Your mother was too good for me but I dragged her down into the gutter with me. Do you still love me, Jean, now that I've told you these things, now that you know I really am no good?'

I kissed him on his cheek in reply.

158

'You understand me much better than your mother,' he said.

We cuddled up close, as we used to do when I was a little girl.

After a while, he rolled over to face the wall and wept. I stood up, feeling sticky-hot, and smoothed my school uniform.

'Tell me what to do, Jean. I wonder if I should see a doctor.'

'Oh yes, Dad. Let's try that.'

Dad was admitted to a dermatology ward. His 'nerves' were aggravating, if not causing, a crippling skin condition; angry sores covered his feet and he couldn't walk. Away from the suffocating tensions of home, he seemed much better.

It was when I visited Dad in hospital that I first experienced a strange sensation. I knew where I was and what I was doing but my head, arms, legs, my whole body and everything around me in the brightly lit ward seemed unreal, as if I was in a dream. After about half an hour this weird dream feeling lifted, but I was left anxiously wondering what was wrong with me.

I absconded from school at break one afternoon when the dream feeling came on strongly, and I spent the rest of the day sitting on my bench in the cemetery. The empty feeling in my stomach told me when it was teatime and I slowly ate my toffee bar.

Last night Dad had woken me up to send me to the 'big bed'. A lot of shouting was going on downstairs and I heard a scream, followed by a silence that was even more worrying than the noise. I'd strained to listen, alert and tense, my head buzzing with questions and fears. The front door slammed. And then a long silence, broken only by the sounds of the night – a tap dripping, a dog's bark, a creak in the floorboards, a distant car, wind against the window. A heavy pain hung darkly at the back of my eyes. It throbbed more violently on each of the several times I got out of bed during the night. But I had to keep getting up and tiptoeing to the landing window to see if Mum was still sitting on the garden wall. In the morning Dad told me how he'd gone for Mum with a stick but ended up *crying at the thought of what he'd been about to do.*

I screwed up my toffee-bar paper and stuffed it into my blazer pocket. The pain behind my eyes was still there. Rubbing my forehead helped to ease it, but I was so tired. Clutching my satchel to my stomach I stared from my bench at the row upon row of headstones. Nobody was in sight; there was nothing to disturb the peace and quiet. The beauty of the white and pink carnations on the nearest grave lifted my spirits. The world might be splintering but here in the healing calmness of this place, with lovely flowers for company, I was safe. A sudden chill in the air broke the spell and reminded me that I had more to think about than pretty flowers. Dad was not normally a violent man although I remembered that once, at Madras Street, he'd bruised Brian with his belt. Recently he'd told me how he feared losing control. Well, supposing he did lose control? What would he do?

And what was I to do? I didn't want to go home. School was unbearable. I was too damn shy to breathe. And now, on top of it all, Dad had told me to decide who I wanted to live with — 'her or me?' How could I even try to choose between them? I hated being fourteen and too young to leave home. Dare I run away? Where to?

The following day I thought my absence at yesterday's last lesson hadn't been noticed when Mr Clark said nothing to me while calling the register. But as the class filed out he stopped me at the door.

'Why weren't you at your last lesson yesterday?'

'I felt funny, sir, so I went home.'

'Why didn't you tell a teacher if you felt unwell?'

'I ... I don't know, sir.'

'You don't know!' he said, placing his hands on his hips, which made his black robe billow out. His dark, beady eyes blazed and the image of a black barrel which had sprung to mind was replaced by that of a mad monk. 'You don't know!' he said again, this time emphasising each world slowly as his head wobbled from side to side. 'Well, you'd better think long and hard about it, hadn't you?'

'Yes, sir.'

'When you're at school, you're in our care. You can't just take off when you please. Can you?'

'No, sir.'

I thought I'd got off lightly but a few days later a letter arrived for my parents asking them to visit the headmaster.

'Do you know what this is about?' Dad asked.

'I think so. You know that dream feeling I told you about? I got it at school and I left early without permission.'

'Well, you shouldn't have,' my mother said, 'but I don't know why he wants us to see him. What can we tell him?'

'Tell him I want to go down into the A2 class,' I said.

Mum was sympathetic to this. She'd seen my diary. I was annoyed that she'd read it without asking, but pleased that she'd shown some interest in what was going on in my life.

A few days later I was sitting opposite the headmaster in his office staring at the carpet.

'I won't bite if you look at me,' he said. I raised my eyes high enough to notice some copies of my reports on his desk. 'I've just had your parents here. They tell me you're unhappy in your class. Is that right?'

'Yes, sir.'

'Why is that?'

'I ... I don't know, sir.' Ironically I was too shy to tell him about my shyness, but I thought he must know about that anyway.

'Would you like to go back down into the A2 form?'

'Oh yes please,' I said, hope rising in me. My friend, Mandy, was in that class.

'I've been looking through your reports,' he said, rustling the papers on his desk, 'and your school work is good. We put you in the highest form because we felt you could cope with the work and we were right. You've no need to worry. You're doing fine.'

I shuffled uncomfortably in my seat.

'Look at it this way. Suppose you were running in a race competing with the best ten runners and you came fifth. You'd

161

have reason to feel more pleased with yourself than if you came first in a race without a good runner. In fact, there'd be no point running in a race without a good runner, would there?'

'No, sir,' I said, my eyes on the carpet.

'Well then, that's why you are in the highest form competing with the brightest children in the school. Do you understand?'

I did not understand. What was the use of being capable of getting good marks in English and History if I wasn't capable of talking to my fellow human beings?

'I ... I don't know, sir,' I said, as the blue circles on the carpet danced and spun dizzily before my eyes.

'Listen, I'll explain it again,' he said, and he launched into an explanation of the runner metaphor, linking it only with academic capabilities and competition.

'Do you understand now?' he asked.

'Yes, sir.'

'So don't worry. There's no problem. I'm pleased with your work. Just keep doing your best, won't you?'

'Yes, sir.'

CHAPTER THIRTEEN

'HAVE YOU DECIDED ABOUT us getting married?' Mike whispered as he leant over and kissed me tenderly. 'I love you.'

A drunken man in a cowboy hat bumped into our table, spilling some of my lager. 'Mike, I've told you I don't want to think about marriage,' I said, mopping the spillage with a beer mat. 'Anyway, how can you say you love me when you don't even know me?'

'Don't know you? I've been going out with you for a year.'

'There's lots of things about me you don't know.'

'Don't tell me, I'll guess. You're married with ten kids and you're a nymphomaniac.'

'Oh, shucks! My secret is out,' I said, covering my face in mock shame and horror. We grinned.

'Do you love me?' Mike asked, becoming serious again.

'I like you a lot as a friend, but ...'

'I'm going to start a new life in New Zealand,' he announced.

'New Zealand?'

'Yes. I've been making enquiries. I did hope we'd get married but if that's not to be, there's nothing to keep me in England.'

'I suppose it's best to stop seeing each other now,' I said, my voice probably conveying less emotion than I was feeling. It's hard to say goodbye to a friend.

'I don't see why,' he said. 'We can go out together till I leave, can't we? As just good friends, I mean. No strings attached.'

'Yes, I … I suppose so,' I said.

Mike proved firm in his intention to emigrate. Despite the 'no strings attached' he kept trying to persuade me to go too, even right up to the time we kissed goodbye, promising to write. I was leading a double life with Mike in that he thought I was still working at Dobson's. He knew nothing about my hospital life. Now he need never know.

Meanwhile, life at the day hospital settled into a routine. After my first week Mr Jordan cancelled my ambulance. He said there seemed no reason why I shouldn't travel on the bus, and I readily agreed. My new doctor was Dr Copeland, though I gathered Dr Shaw was in overall charge of the treatment of day patients.

Mr Jordan showed me into the little office on the first floor and introduced me to Dr Copeland, a stocky dark-haired man sitting at a desk by the window.

'Sit down,' Dr Copeland said to me. 'I'm just reading your case notes.'

I sat opposite the doctor at his desk, while Mr Jordan sat by the door.

Dr Copeland looked up from reading and asked with a grin, 'Am I going to hell because I'm an atheist?'

I took it that he hadn't meant this as a serious question so I didn't bother to answer. He began doodling on a notepad which had some red lettering printed across the top and, in idle curiosity, I strained my eyes to make out what it said. I managed to read: 'MOGADON – THE MARK OF GOOD SLEEP'.

'Well? Am I going to hell?'

'How do I know where you're going?' I said, feeling irritable.

He glanced across at Mr Jordan, and they laughed.

I wondered if they thought I was a religious fanatic, though I couldn't see how questioning and losing my beliefs could fit me for that category – quite the opposite I would have thought. It didn't take me long to decide that nothing was being meant unkindly and, as I tried to describe my sadness and confusion to them, I discovered that I hadn't lost the ability to laugh at myself.

Therapy at the day hospital was usually led by two student nurses and took the form of group games like the one organised by Sue on my first day, and activities such as handicrafts, dominoes and draughts. Some of the day patients, myself included, were sent to join the in-patients at the OT block in the main hospital for a few hours a day.

In summer I was taken out occasionally with some in-patients from the OT block to the nearby town of Otley. I became immune to the stares of passers-by as we ambled along in twos, a nurse in front of the crocodile and two more keeping watch from behind. As we passed a fruit stall in the market, one of the long-stay patients, Amy, casually picked up a shiny red apple and began eating it. The nurses didn't notice but an irate assistant did.

'Hey! You! What d'yer think yer doin'?'

Amy wandered on, obliviously, munching her apple.

'She's a thief!' the fat woman in a white apron screeched.

If the passers-by hadn't been staring at us before, they were now.

The nurse from the back of the line rushed up to Amy. 'What *are* you playing at? Give it back and apologise.'

She frogmarched Amy to the assistant on the stall. Amy took another bite of the apple before placing it among the others on display.

'Do yer think I can sell that now? Do yer?' This was addressed to the nurse, since Amy didn't seem to know or care what the fuss was about.

'I'm really sorry,' the nurse said, unzipping her purse.

After that, we shuffled along a bit further, while the nurse gave Amy a long-winded sermon about not taking things that didn't belong to her.

'Buy your Beatles pictures here,' a man with a Beatles haircut who looked at least in his forties announced. 'Get your big colour photos of the Fab Four.'

'The Beatles split up last year,' a young man in a 'The Who' T-shirt informed him as he sauntered past.

'So what?' the man on the stall called after him.

'Let go. Move on.'

I stopped to watch a group of mini-skirted teenage girls who were dancing by the side of this stall and singing 'All You Need Is Love'. I guessed some of us who grew up in the Beatles era would never be able to let go and move on. A part of me longed to join in the fun and be just another ordinary teenager again.

'C'mon, you. Stop dawdling,' the nurse admonished me.

No going back.

On another trip to Otley, a nurse praised me profusely, in earshot of a shop assistant and people in the queue, for counting out the correct amount of money to pay for a bar of chocolate. I wanted to protest that I wasn't mentally retarded, but perhaps this would have been a tactless remark to make in front of the group of patients I was with that day. This random mixing of two sets of patients with quite different needs, the 'mentally ill' and the 'mentally handicapped' (as they were then called) for want of better terminology, seemed to me to be not good for either set of patients, or the staff.

I remembered from my stay as an in-patient the many instances I'd seen or experienced where staff talked down to patients. I wondered if, in my case, my shy, passive behaviour contributed to this. On the other hand, it did seem a no-win situation because our reactions to humiliating circumstances, whether of anger, rebellion or withdrawal, could be interpreted by staff as evidence of 'mental illness' no matter how justifiable our responses might be. Rebellious patients could be broken into submission through stronger drugs, more ECT and psychological cruelty, but there was an equally high price to be paid by those of us who accepted the psychiatric view of ourselves as 'sick' and co-operated with treatment. Brainwashing techniques, aided by both physical and psychological means, at a time when a person is already weak, unhappy and vulnerable, can be extremely effective. Although a part of my drugged, assaulted mind was sometimes critical about what was going on, I still, for the most part, quietly complied.

I often passed a door at OT that bore the label 'GROUP THERAPY'. What went on in this room? Were interesting discussions organised? Were patients encouraged to form a kind of self-help group, perhaps? I felt curiously optimistic when told to join the group of patients in that room one afternoon.

The patients inside, however, seemed severely disturbed or drugged out of their senses. The woman sitting next to me kept tugging at her hair while moaning softly to herself. There were about seven of us, including the therapist, a slim, blonde girl of about nineteen who wore beetle-shaped earrings. I wondered what we were going to do. The man sitting opposite me didn't seem interested in doing anything except masturbating.

'Let's first get to know each other's names,' said the therapist, who was sitting on a chair in the middle of the group with a pile of newspapers in her lap. 'I'm Christine.' She went round the group getting our names and wrote them down on a notepad. Then she gave each of us a newspaper. And not just the tabloids; mine was a 'quality' newspaper. The mystery deepened. Whatever were we going to do? I would have liked to join a group where we could discuss issues arising from newspaper articles; something to help my bruised mind to think again. Being encouraged to participate in group discussion might also have helped me overcome shyness. But, no, this group had definitely not been put together for a discussion of current affairs.

'Jack! Stop eating your paper!' Christine said to an elderly, dazed-looking man who was busily engaged in chewing the corner of a page.

Christine glanced round at us and clapped her hands for attention. 'Can you see where the pages are numbered?' she asked. 'Everyone have a look at the numbers at the bottom of the pages. Can you all see them? Right, now listen carefully.

These pages have been mixed up, so what does that mean? It means that the numbers don't follow on in the correct order. Let's see who will be the quickest at putting their newspaper into the correct order. Find page number one first, and then page numbers two, three, four, five and so on. Put the pages so that the numbers run on. Spread them out on the floor if you like. Do you all understand what you've to do? OK? Ready. Steady. GO!'

Everyone began sorting out their papers except the masturbator, the paper-eater and myself. I didn't move because I was preoccupied with something else, something more important.

Ignoring the other two dissenters, Christine addressed me: 'Come on, Jean. You understand, don't you?'

Caught off guard, I almost blurted out, 'No. I don't understand.'

What I didn't understand was how, merely by confiding in a psychiatrist in my teens that I was confused about religion and disillusioned with life, I had got myself into all this.

My therapy routine included three mornings a week at the Office Skills class but, as when I was an in-patient, I was too drugged and unmotivated to benefit. I plodded through shorthand exercises taking in more of my depressing surroundings than of the symbols I was supposed to be learning. As far as learning shorthand goes, I was wasting my time. But about human misery, for what good it would do me, I was learning a lot.

There was Nina, a shy-looking teenager with long black hair and large brown eyes, who sought the help of Mrs Taylor, the typing teacher, to explain what her Ward Sister meant by describing her as 'inadequate'. Nina was wanting to leave home and get a flat after her discharge from hospital.

'Sister says I'll never be able to cope in a flat because I'm inadequate. What does "inadequate" mean?' Nina asked the kindly Mrs Taylor, who floundered while trying to answer her.

Earlier that morning a nurse had told a group of us at the

day hospital that the reason we were patients and 'different' from people like herself was because we had a 'weaker personality', which made us unable to cope with the everyday anxieties of life.

The worst thing about being constantly taught that you're 'sick', 'inadequate' or have a 'weaker personality' is that you might eventually come to believe it. And the worst thing about coming to believe it is that this will help it become true.

I made friends with Wendy at OT, a pretty sixteen-year-old, who was having problems coming to terms with her abortion. She was a patient in Thornville Ward. One day we were talking at tea break in the cloakroom, where it was a little more private than the corridors and hall.

'My psychiatrist says I've to forget about the abortion,' she told me. 'My baby was taken from my womb and murdered but I'm supposed to forget that happened. How can I?' She finished her cigarette and lit another. 'God, I'm chain-smoking again but that's the least of my problems.'

A man wandered up to us trying to cadge a cigarette. We recoiled as we smelt his breath. He was puffing nervously at an over-smoked tab end.

'Go away! We're having a private conversation,' Wendy told him.

Head down, looking as if he'd no pride left, he turned and moved dejectedly away.

'Oh what the hell, take it, have them all,' Wendy said, running after him with the packet.

He pushed the cigarette she lit for him into his mouth and we watched him shuffling away, his shirt hanging out of his trousers.

'Silly old bugger,' Wendy said, 'but oh, Jean, isn't life sad for people like him?'

I nodded in agreement.

'Now what was I saying? Oh yes,' she said, 'my psychiatrist says I've to forget I was pregnant and he says I'm the same girl as I was before ... before it happened. But I'm not the same, am I, Jean? How can I ever be the same? I'm not innocent any more.'

Tears sprang to her big blue eyes, smudging her mascara and running down her pink, dimpled cheeks, as she wept for lost innocence.

And there was Cathy, a pale, thin young woman who had been a teacher. She stood at the front of the typing class holding a cactus plant from the windowsill and proceeded to give us a lecture on it. Our botany lesson ended abruptly when Mrs Taylor came in and asked her what on earth she was doing.

Cathy stopped lecturing mid-sentence, cactus plant still in hand, and looked thoughtful. 'What am I doing? Well, I'm obviously mad as a hatter, aren't I? I suppose I'm pretending I'm still a teacher because that time of my life was better than now.' She broke down and sobbed. Mrs Taylor put a comforting arm around her shoulder and gently led her to a seat at a typewriter. 'I'd do Miss Compton proud now,' Cathy said, half laughing, half crying.

'Miss Compton?'

'Yeah. I'm talking about Lena Compton's drama group. That's the drama group I used to be in and the drama group I'd still be in if I wasn't round the twist here in High Royds instead.'

'But you're getting better, Catherine dear. You'll be able to go back to the drama group, and perhaps even back to teaching, when you're well again, don't you think?'

'No, that's not possible. It's all over now. Can't you see? Everything is finished, spoilt, changed, broken ...'

The cactus plant had been left balancing precariously on the edge of Mrs Taylor's desk at the front of the class. I watched, half expecting it to emphasise Cathy's words by toppling over and crashing to the floor.

LOOKING BACK 7

THE BEATLES WERE COMING to Bradford. On Friday 9th October 1964 the Fab Four would be starting their UK tour right on our doorstep, appearing at the Gaumont Theatre. Of course we had to go. I hadn't been out with Sylvia, Carrie and Julia for a while, but we'd managed to save up for tickets costing 10s.6d, expensive in those days.

I couldn't wait to get out of my school uniform that night and into my red skirt and domino-spotted blouse. My new suspender belt dug into my stomach even though I was stick-thin. Nylon stockings always made my legs itch, but I was getting used to them. I felt really grown up, especially with my lightly-padded bra making the most of what I hadn't got. I back-combed my hair, brushed blue sparkly shadow onto my eyelids and painted my lips 'sugar-pink'.

Before the show started, the packed theatre was buzzing. The moment they came on stage, hysteria gripped the audience. Beatlemania, the papers called it. Everyone was standing on their seats, yelling and screaming like crazy. My mates were already doing the same. I clambered up onto my seat and we screamed ourselves hoarse. I couldn't make out who was shouting what in the deafening din, but I knew Carrie would be yelling 'John', Julia 'George' and, for Sylvia and me, it had to be 'Paul'. We could neither see nor hear the group that we'd paid so much money for, but the show was fantastic. It must have been.

When it was over, we hung about in the dark cobbled alley at the back of the theatre, along with a crowd of other hopefuls, waiting for a glimpse of the Beatles leaving by the back door.

Policemen shooed us away. My brand new stockings were laddered from ankle to knee but that didn't matter. We roamed the night-time streets of town, arms linked, singing Beatles songs at the top of our voices.

What a come-down after the Beatles show to be back in my school uniform, back in the role of a shy, quiet schoolgirl. Oh, if only I'd stayed at my other school with my friends. We'd be sitting at our desks now, whispering and giggling behind our hands, sharing our feelings about that special event.

I decided it was the situation which had already been created in my class at Rossfields that made it impossible for me to change things. In Geography, a note was passed to me, which read:

Dear Jean,
 Sally and I have decided not to let you come in our team in Gym. Nobody likes you in this class.
 Joyce and Sally.

PS: Send us this note back or we'll smash your face after school tonight

It seemed my only chance of breaking the shyness barrier would be with people who didn't already know me, so I resolved to leave school as soon as it became legally possible.

I was scribbling on my notebook in a music lesson, working out how long before I could leave Rossfields if I didn't stay on to take GCE O levels. Miss Barr, the music teacher, wasn't paying any attention to what I was doing. She was a lively, young-looking woman with curly red hair and twinkling green eyes. When the class started altering the words of a song we were singing, she even joined in herself with the fun. At my previous school with my old friends I'd have been enjoying joining in too. There, I'd been caned for talking, laughing and clowning in class. Here, I could only observe the scene with

172

discomfort through that invisible barrier of shyness, which separated me from my classmates as effectively as stout prison walls.

The laughter got louder till the class was in uproar. Our form teacher, Mr Clark, was attempting to take an English lesson in the classroom next door. He strode into Miss Barr's room and, with eyebrows that formed one bushy line right across his forehead, demanded to know what was going on.

Next day, after calling the register, Mr Clark said, 'Stand up those of you who fooled about in yesterday's music lesson.'

At first no one moved. Then Bobby Spencer stood up. 'Come on now. Everybody stand up. It was all of us.' Chairs scraped as pupils stood up. 'Is everyone standing?' Bobby asked, looking around. 'Come on, Carol and Daphne, you too. And you, Stephen, don't pretend it wasn't you as well.' Then Bobby's eyes fell on me and he said nothing. More chairs scraped as more pupils stood up until everyone was standing. Except me.

How I wanted to stand up, to be like the others, but I had not, as everyone knew, been making a noise, so I remained self-consciously seated. It is a strange feeling indeed to be the only one seated in the middle of a room full of about thirty people. I felt isolated, vulnerable and very small. Gulliver in the Land of Giants.

I continued to count the days to leaving Rossfields. The long months limped on, dragging me with them. When I felt it would never end, when I felt I could stand no more, I caught a glimpse of my fifteenth birthday on the horizon. Getting there. Despite my problems at school and at home I did well in my mock GCE O Levels. I failed abysmally in Maths and Cookery but achieved good results in my favourite subjects of English Language, Literature, Scripture Knowledge and History. No way could I stay on an extra year or more to take my exams. Any job, no matter how boring, would surely be more bearable than school.

More miserable months passed. Not long now. I was glad

I'd been born in time. Mandy, being a few months younger than me, had to stay on at school longer. She was off sick when I left.

No more school. Fifteen. Old enough to leave Rossfields. At the end of my last day there, while the other school-leavers were hugging, weeping and saying their goodbyes, I buttoned my gabardine raincoat, slipped out of the school gates and headed down the road. The relief I'd expected to feel didn't come until later. I dragged my feet as if I'd got weights tied to them. One glance back. And then eyes down on the blurring grey pavement. No one to say goodbye to.

She finished school at 15 but did not take any exams.

Dr Prior

CHAPTER FOURTEEN

CAROLINE HAD AN OLD worn pop record called 'The Heart of a Teenage Girl', which she played over and over again on the record player at the day hospital. Amidst clicks and scratches, Craig Douglas's voice filled the room with laments about the brevity of the teen years.

'I've missed out on an ordinary teenage life,' Caroline said wistfully. 'I'd love to go to places where ordinary teenagers go. Do you go to discos, Jean?'

'Yes.'

'Oh, tell me about them. Describe in detail what it's like there. Please,' she begged, her eyes shining in anticipation. I felt uncomfortable. Here was someone who was envying my life, a life I was so dissatisfied with but which, in comparison to hers, was indeed a life I ought to be counting my blessings for.

'Go on, describe a disco to me,' Caroline persisted.

So I told her about the coloured, flashing lights, the noise, the dancing. I didn't want to make Caroline's sense of missing out on something harder to bear, so I tried not to make them sound as exciting and wonderful as she seemed to think they were. But I didn't say that discos are places where sometimes teenagers become screwed up with drugs and get their lives ruined. That's what happens in mental hospitals, too, I thought cynically, so Caroline will know enough about that.

'Oh, I'd love to go,' Caroline said again, with more enthusiasm than ever after my description.

The following Monday Caroline was not at the hospital. She had run away at the weekend, presumably in search of that 'ordinary teenage life' she'd never had.

My thoughts kept returning to Caroline. Would she be exploited, raped, murdered? She was so vulnerable, anything could happen. And was it partly my fault for telling her about discos? My worries and fears for her safety increased with each passing day.

I tried to avoid sitting with Geoff at lunchtime because it was true, as Sue had said, that he was frequently sick. I groaned inwardly when he sat beside me with his plate.

'Did you know...' he began as he shovelled in huge mouthfuls of mashed potato.

'Geoff, don't eat so quickly or you'll be sick,' I pleaded.

'Did you know,' he began again, 'my mother tried to abort me.'

Marlene raised her eyebrows. She was a young woman in her late twenties who was always feisty despite medication that made her drowsy. 'It's a pity she didn't succeed,' she said unkindly.

'I wasn't speaking to you. Speak when you're spoken to.'

He turned to me again. 'Yes, it's true. When she was pregnant with me she tried to have an abortion. But it didn't work.'

He was looking at me as if expecting a reply but I didn't know what to say.

'She tried to abort me!' Geoff said again, pausing from eating to bang his fork on the plate in a way that reminded me of my brother.

'Did she?' I said lamely.

'Yes. That's why I'm like I am.'

Marlene said, 'What do you mean, Geoff? Are you saying you're brain damaged because she tried to abort you or did she try to abort you because she knew you was going to be brain damaged?'

Before Geoff could respond to this, an eerie scream filled the air, followed by a crash, and Vera was writhing on the floor.

177

'Mr Jordan, come quick! Vera's having one of her fits,' somebody yelled. Mr Jordan bent over Vera who smacked him and kicked him with her flailing arms and legs. When she came to, tears were rolling down her face as she looked around in a daze.

Vera was a friendly, jovial woman in her forties who caught the same bus as me on the three days a week that she attended the day hospital, and on these journeys my shyness with her had gradually disappeared. She invited me to her house for tea one Thursday, and this became a weekly occurrence.

'You *will* still come for tea today, won't you?' Vera asked me almost as soon as she opened her eyes.

'Yes, of course I will, if you feel well enough to want me to.'

'Oh yes, I'm all right now,' she said. 'I *so* much look forward to you coming.'

Still dazed, she was trying to light the wrong end of a cigarette and smiled when she realised this.

'Seeing me like you did just now hasn't put you off me, has it?' she asked anxiously.

'Don't be daft, of course it hasn't,' I said.

Although Vera behaved on the surface like a cheerful, extrovert woman, she seemed very lonely and unsure of herself.

After tea at Vera's that evening, I dutifully swallowed my medication. Vera opened various plastic containers and filled her palm with an assortment of pills. Her ten-year-old daughter, Jill, came to sit on a pouffe in front of her mother who, with an upward sweeping movement of her palm, caught all the pills in her mouth and swallowed them down without a drink in one gulp.

'That was a little trick I do to amuse Jill,' Vera explained.

I wondered if it would have a bad effect on Jill, growing up seeing pills swallowed like sweets, but, worse still, Vera said that when she told a nurse at the hospital how she sometimes felt unable to cope when Jill was boisterous, the nurse told her to give Jill a small amount of crushed Largactil to 'quieten her

178

down'.

Later that evening, when Vera's husband was at the pub and Jill was in bed, we got talking about Caroline's disappearance.

'I'm worried about Caroline,' I confided.

'Oh, don't worry about her,' Vera said. 'She's tougher than you think, Jean. People like her are born survivors.'

I doubted strongly that Caroline could have learnt in a mental institution the kind of survival skills she would need in the outside world.

'Remember Georgina telling us how she ran away from a mental hospital when she was Caroline's age?' Vera said, still trying to reassure me. 'Well, no great harm came to her, did it?'

'No, not from running away,' I agreed.

Georgina was a day patient who often talked to Vera and me about the mental institutions she'd been in over the last forty years. Her stories chronicled the dark history of the psychiatric profession. She told of padded cells, ice baths, insulin treatment, ECT without anaesthetic, having to eat with wooden spatulas … And now Georgina had become the 'star patient' of students' training classes. Somehow, through it all, she had been able to retain a strong sense of humour, but every now and then she tried to kill herself, her last attempt being only a few weeks ago.

'It's not easy to die,' Georgina told me. 'I haven't got it right yet, but one day I'll succeed.'

Georgina lived with her married daughter. She came to and from the hospital by ambulance as she was agoraphobic. Vera and I encouraged her to come with us for a cup of tea at the little café a few minutes' walk away from the hospital drive. She managed to do this several times, but as soon as we left the hospital gates she would turn white and cling nervously to us.

'I'm scared of people,' she said on her way back from the café one day. 'Not of people like you two, or the other patients, but of all the people outside.'

'And they're probably scared to death of us,' Vera said with

179

a smile.

'Do you think people outside can tell just by looking at me that I'm different from them?' she asked touchingly. 'Would you know I was a patient, Jean, if you saw me in the street and didn't know me?'

'Not unless you were going about wearing a badge that says "HIGH ROYDS MENTAL HOSPITAL" on it,' I said.

Georgina laughed but she kept a tight grip on my hand as we walked back to the hospital. It was true that no one would have known just by looking that this woman, who always took the trouble to wear make-up and dress smartly, had been in and out of mental hospitals throughout most of her life. That she could function only *inside* the mental hospital world after all those years of being a patient didn't surprise me. What did surprise me was that she could function at all; that something positive in her personality had managed to survive intact through all the years of treatment.

A few weeks after Caroline's disappearance, the police brought her back. She had hitchhiked to London, spent some nights sleeping rough in a park, and been to an all-nighter disco. Thinner but starry-eyed, she described the disco in glowing terms and then went on to tell us about the cold, dark nights in the park with strange men who 'wrap themselves in newspapers and sleep on benches'. She didn't sound too sad to be back 'home', and spoke as if she was telling us about an enjoyable holiday. I supposed for her it had been just that. A kind of holiday when, at least for a while, she had been transported away from the hospital world.

Some weeks later Caroline was found to be pregnant though it was thought that this might have occurred since her return to hospital. Either way it didn't make any difference. An abortion brought a swift solution. Poor Caroline. Barely out of her teens, she had lived so much and yet so little.

Like Caroline, I, too, was transported away from the hospital world for a while. This was when Mandy and I went for a fortnight's holiday, staying in Belgium and visiting Holland and France. I had a reserve of savings in the bank from my working days and this seemed as good a reason as any to draw out some money.

When Mandy and I applied for our passports we got the ten-year type, planning to do more travelling in the future. We said we wanted to visit exotic places, see other cultures, meet interesting people, but for me all this excited talking was just a tenuous dream. Drugged, drowsy and depressed as I was, diagnosed as sick and submerged in a life centred on a mental hospital, any dream of future *living* seemed as unreal as the dream of the old woman with wrinkled stockings falling about her ankles who tugged at my sleeve as we passed in one of the dismal hospital corridors. 'I must tell you this,' she said, with saliva dribbling down her chin and on to her shapeless floral-print dress. 'I'm really a princess and will soon be crowned Queen of England.'

I couldn't imagine going abroad without writing about it, so I packed a notebook-cum-diary along with my pills. Sitting in our hotel bedroom in Ostend, staring at the blank page and chewing my pen, I realised with dismay that even writing had become just another difficult and tiring chore.

I watched Mandy, who was sitting next to me on our peach quilted bed, writing enthusiastically about our holiday so far. She handed it to me to read, then I copied what she'd written into my diary, making the excuse that I was too tired to do my own writing. I did the same for my postcards. We'd been to the same places, done the same things, so her description would suffice, I told myself. What did it matter?

But later that night, staring through the window up at the dark Belgian sky, I asked myself when and why had I relinquished the ability to live; to feel, laugh, cry, and to write? Of course it mattered! What was I doing? Living by proxy?

Our hotel was described in the brochure as 'situated in the heart of the night life'. In a stiflingly hot and crowded disco, the young man I'd been dancing with for most of the evening suggested we go for a walk. After searching the crowd for

Mandy and eventually finding her locked in the arms of a continental Romeo, I arranged to meet her back at the disco later. She disentangled herself from her man long enough to agree to this. So off Claude and I went, hand in hand, to stroll around the streets, breathing in the cool night air.

Claude was tall, handsome, polite and charming. He was used to speaking only in French so, not surprisingly, had a few problems understanding my English, working-class, northern accent.

'Slow down, slow down. I am trying to listen to you, translate what you are saying into French in my head, and then I have to translate my thoughts back into English so that I can answer you. It is not easy.'

Perhaps the cheap wine I'd been drinking in the disco was taking effect as I began to relax and enjoy myself. It turned midnight but the streets throbbed with life, and music from the bars and discos filled the air.

We turned into a quaint little bar where Claude bought me a gin and tonic. I learnt he was a schoolteacher with an interest in history, politics and current affairs. He asked my opinion on Britain's entry into the Common Market. How abysmally little I knew about *anything* other than a mental hospital, I realised with shame. I wasn't knowledgeable enough in current affairs to have an intelligent opinion, but I bluffed it, feigning the language problem whenever I got really stuck.

After leaving the bar, we walked to the sea front and watched the outline of a ship, all bright lights looming up out of darkness, as it approached the harbour. There, beside the water, he kissed me passionately and made bold sexual advances, but when I asked him to stop he did so immediately.

'Please forgive me,' he said. 'You, Jean, are different from other English girls I have met. You are very sweet.'

And you, Claude, are a typical sweet-talking guy, I thought.

'Am I allowed to kiss?' he asked ever so politely. *'S'il vous plaît?'*

I nodded. 'Yes, but no more than kissing. Do you understand?'

'*Oui, je comprends. Merci.*'

We kissed, and then went to another bar. As I sipped my drink, I glanced at my watch. 'The time! Oh, goodness, look at the time!'

It was too late to meet Mandy at the disco, so I tried to find the hotel. Claude insisted on staying with me, though I would have been happier now to walk these strange, brightly lit foreign streets alone, free from having to make the effort to talk. I was embarrassed that I couldn't even remember the name of my hotel, let alone the address. My sense of direction, seemingly worsened by ECT, left much to be desired, so we wandered the maze of streets for a long time.

At last I recognised a building near my hotel and found my way from there. After a lingering goodbye kiss and cuddle with Claude, I went inside and padded softly along the carpeted corridors, trying not to wake anyone. Fortunately, I could remember our room number. A slit of light showed from the edges of our door.

'Where the hell have you been?' Mandy was sitting up in bed, running her fingers through thick, black curls, her dark eyes flashing. 'Look at the time!'

'You sound like an angry parent,' I said, grinning.

'Well, I've been worried about you,' Mandy said with such feeling that I immediately felt guilty.

'I'm sorry, Mandy,' I said, sitting beside her on the bed. 'I didn't realise you'd be worried about me.'

She looked as if she was about to cry. 'How could I *not* worry? I'm your friend, remember? Friends do worry about each other, don't they?'

'I … I'm really sorry, Mandy,' I said again, deeply moved by her obvious concern. I remembered how I used to worry about her, but she'd grown up a lot since then. I should have grown up too, but I didn't seem to be making a very good job of it.

What do I remember most about that holiday? Was it the thrill of travelling by plane for the first time? Or the adventure of being in other countries? Did I really see that view of Paris from the top of the Eiffel Tower, those winding cobbled streets in Brussels, the scenic beauty of the Dutch countryside dotted here and there with quaint windmills? These things miraculously appeared on my photographs when my film was developed, but they had hardly touched me at all.

So what did I see? I saw hippies living in dirty, smelly barges on a river in Amsterdam. In the late sixties and early seventies, Amsterdam was known as 'Hippysville'. I stared through a barge window watching a hippy couple and their baby until the youth stuck two fingers up at me. I couldn't blame him, of course, for I was being terribly nosey. I wandered back round the corner of Dam Square where there were more hippies, a large gathering of them, sitting around on the ground. Some of them looked 'together' but others, with their bland expressions and vacant eyes, looked spaced out on drugs. It seemed to me that the 'alternative' society had as many flaws, pitfalls and hypocrisy as a conventional lifestyle and I suspected that many hippies led lives as barren as my own. But, perhaps because I thought they too were rejecting something, I felt drawn to them.

Holiday over, it was back to England, back to High Royds, back to the familiar hospital routine. Caroline was worried because the staff on her ward had threatened her with a leucotomy for being 'aggressive and cheeky'. A leucotomy, I learned, was a brain operation carried out by a neurosurgeon, which involves making a cut in the front area of the brain. This operation is irreversible and large mental hospitals, like High Royds, all had their share of the unfortunate recipients of 'unsuccessful' leucotomies among their cabbage patches. Of course, there is a big difference between threatening to leucotomise a patient and actually doing it, but if the threat is taken seriously (and is there not every reason to take it seriously?) then the fear is very real.

'Jean, do you think I need a leucotomy?' Caroline asked as we walked in the hospital grounds before dinner. With head hung down, hands in her duffle coat pockets, she was kicking a stone along the path. 'If they want to do it, should I let them?'

No, no, a thousand times no, I felt like yelling. But if 'they' decided they wanted to do it to her, then I wondered what kind of choice poor Caroline would have.

'I don't think I'd let them even if it meant I had to kill myself to stop them,' she said, giving the stone a harder kick as she answered my unspoken question.

Geoff, too, was concerned about choices. He had just returned to the day hospital after spending some time as an in-patient. Standing in the dinner queue he kept asking, 'Do we get a choice?'

Everybody ignored him except Marlene who suddenly exploded. 'For heaven's sake, shut up, Geoff. You're getting on my nerves. *Do we get a choice?* What are you talking about?'

'We got a choice for dinner on the ward,' he said.

'Well, you're not on that ward now and we've never had a choice here,' she snapped.

A few minutes later Geoff was asking again, 'Do we get a choice?' but this time I noticed a smile playing on Marlene's lips.

'Yes, Geoff, you do get a choice,' she said, with a chuckle. 'You either eat it or you don't.'

I smiled to myself, but then remembered Lynette, the little hunch-backed woman in Thornville Ward, who hadn't even been given that choice.

LOOKING BACK 8

'*I DON'T KNOW HOW I*'ll *be able to get a good job with no O levels,*' *I said to my mother.*

'*You don't need those fancy things. Why don't you get a job at the Fisk television factory like Edna Wright's daughter? Now, that's a sensible, down-to-earth job.*'

'*I don't want to work in a factory.*'

'*I thought you'd turn your nose up at that, Lady Jane. When I was your age I worked in a mill. I don't suppose you'd like to work in a mill either, would you?*'

'*You're dead right, I wouldn't,*' *I said.*

'*I don't understand you,*' *she said in exasperation.* '*The mill was good enough for me and for my father before me and for his father before him. Why do you have to be so different? Even Edna's lass doesn't think a factory job's beneath her, and I always thought she was too big for her boots. What's wrong with working in a factory?*'

'*Nowt's wrong with working in a factory. I don't think it's beneath me. But I'm not interested in what Edna's daughter or anyone else is doing. That's up to them, but I am ME.*'

I stormed out of the room, slamming the door.

Upstairs sitting on my bed I thought things over. Perhaps I should go for an interview at Fisk's after all. Perhaps it was as good a job as any that was open to me. At least it would be an opportunity for a brand-new start, I told myself, trying to quell my apprehension. This time I would have to force myself to talk from the beginning. At all costs I had to avoid creating the same situation I'd been in at Rossfields.

'*Please, God, don't let me mess up my brand-new start,*' *I*

186

prayed on my knees on the eve of my launching into the World of Work.

My factory job consisted of brushing grease onto a metal rotor, slotting it into a part destined to fit somewhere inside a television, adding a few screws, wires and metal fixtures, two blobs of hot solder, then passing it on to the next person. A two-minute job which a monkey could be trained to do. Repeated over two hundred times per day: more than a thousand times a week. In less than a week I was struggling to bear boredom so excruciating it was like a physical pain. But my mother was pleased that I had given up my 'high-and-mighty ideas' and settled for a 'sensible down-to-earth job'. If only I'd kicked harder in protest. Instead I tried, God knows how hard I tried, to conform to the role that was expected of me. And in so doing I almost destroyed myself.

On the assembly line I sat next to Joanne Foster who, like me, was a fifteen-year-old school leaver in her first job. After a few days, a pattern was establishing with me saying nothing all day while Joanne and the others laughed and talked. Rossfields loomed large. I must talk. I must talk. I must.

I felt uncomfortably warm, warmer, hot, now stifling hot. My clothes were sticking to me as if sweat was seeping from every pore in my body. My heart was beating loud and fast, and I was shaking, literally shaking, as if a giant, quivering jelly had been planted in my insides. Could I do it? Dare I? I'd simply got to.

Ignore the shy feelings and they'll go away, I tried telling myself. But they did not go away. Well, let them wash over me, it doesn't matter. Talk NOW. My heart beat faster; my stomach churned. The only dialogue I was participating in was the one going on inside me. Yes, I can talk. I can. I'll speak to Joanne now. I must. I will ... And I nearly burst with the effort of trying to speak.

For part of the day, pop music blared out through speakers. My favourite songs at that time often reflected my mood of hopeful longing. I took to heart the words of the Animals when they sang 'We've Gotta Get Out of This Place'. Oh God, yes, surely there was a better life than this. I also loved to hear Donovan singing 'Catch the Wind'. 'Mr Tambourine Man' sung by the Byrds was another of my favourites; even better than Bob Dylan's version.

The other girls would sing to the songs that came on. If only I wasn't too shy to join in with the talking and singing, my boredom with the job would lessen. How I hated my shyness since it infiltrated into every part of my life and made other problems, such as the boredom, much worse.

One day I was again trying to find courage to join in talking with Joanne and the others, when they lowered their voices. After conversing in whispers for a while, Joanne turned to me and asked loudly: 'Why don't yer talk to us, Jean? We all want to know.' The chatter around me stopped. Everyone was watching me intently.

'Aren't we good enough for yer?' Joanne asked.

The question hurt as if a wet knife had been dipped in salt and twisted inside a still-open wound. In all those months of longing to leave Rossfields, my hopes had been pinned on things being different at work. I wasn't at Rossfields now. The place was different. The girls were different. But I was just the same.

'Are yer deaf as well as dumb?' Joanne asked. The other girls giggled. 'We want to know why yer don't talk.'

Why didn't I talk? All I knew was how much I wanted to, how much I tried and how miserably I'd failed. Now I wanted to go off alone somewhere to cry out the hurt and disappointment in myself. I was looking down at a blob of solder on my bench as if it had assumed tremendous importance. Joanne was still waiting for an answer. I forced myself to meet her gaze. 'I ... I do talk,' I said feebly. Joanne raised her eyebrows to the ceiling and everyone collapsed into fits of giggles.

After this, it would have been no harder for me to jump over the moon than to talk. If I couldn't do it at first when Joanne had been friendly towards me, how could I do it now?

'Open yer mouth,' Joanne said, turning to me one day. 'Go on, open it. Or I'll burn yer with this.' She picked up her soldering iron.

'Get lost!'

'I saw it! I saw it!' she exclaimed, amidst peals of laughter. 'We thought yer hadn't got a tongue.' She stood up and shouted: 'Hey, come and look, everyone! She's got a tongue!'

Even the girls facing me on a different assembly line were staring at me and joining in the laughter. I was drowning in a sea of smiling faces all around me.

While my shyness with colleagues seemed unmovable, I improved at small talk with lads who 'chatted me up'. I palled up with my old friend Jackie again, and hung about town till late every night.

Some boys who tagged on to us one night took us down an alley to show us where Baxter, a sixteen-year-old gang leader, had been knifed.

'It was just here. I'm standing on the exact spot,' said a greasy-haired youth who was wearing a black leather jacket with a skull and crossbones painted in luminous white on the back. 'He was stabbed here in the ribs and you should've seen the blood oozing out,' he went on, his eyes shining coldly. 'Wish I'd got a torch to show you the bloodstains.' He turned his back to us and bent down in the shadows. All we could see was the skull and crossbones moving and gleaming in the darkness.

'Is ... is he dead?' I asked. My memory of Baxter, a handsome, tall guy with a 'little boy lost' look in his eyes, was merging with the skeleton skull bobbing about in front of me.

'Not yet, I don't think. He's in hospital and he's dying.'

'But why?' I asked in dismay. 'Why did it happen?'

He shrugged his shoulders. 'Who knows or cares? Hey, you didn't fancy him, did you?'

'Get lost!'

Jackie and one of the boys started 'necking' and the rest of them walked away. All except the boy with the cold shining

189

eyes who had located the 'exact spot'.

'Well, what are we waiting for?' he asked, grabbing hold of me. 'You're a real cutie.' I disliked him so much that I instinctively stepped back.

'What are you doing?' a voice boomed out. Startled, we all looked round to see two policemen who shone their torches on us.

'Necking,' replied Cold Eyes. 'Ain't no law against that, is there?'

One of the policemen addressed me sternly: 'You're too young to be roaming around town at night.'

'No I'm not,' I retorted. 'I'm fifteen.'

That night in bed I thought about Joe Baxter. It seemed such a depressing, senseless way for a sixteen-year-old life to end. Nobody seemed to know what the fight had been about. Even Cold Eyes, who'd been there at the time and knew all the gory details, hadn't known or cared why it had started. He was more interested in the 'How?' than the 'Why?'

A hundred WHYS were pounding my brain. Dismayed by the things I saw in newspapers, on TV, and at night in the rough streets and bars of Bradford, I was becoming increasingly disillusioned at the seeming emptiness and superficiality of everything. The talks I had with Jackie when there were just the two of us were as refreshing as a tumbler full of cool, clear spring water. We took ourselves so seriously, moralising smugly about the state of the world and the pressures placed on us poor teenagers of today, then we would see the funny side and laugh at ourselves till our sides ached. But the only boys we met seemed as shallow as Cold Eyes. And then we would all use so many words to say absolutely nothing.

I stopped thinking I could help my parents or Brian with their problems; I knew now I needed all the strength I possessed to cope with my 'growing pains'. I felt alienated from my family and wanted to be in the house as little as possible.

I decided it was time to take stock of myself; to think about what I was doing and where I was going. But this kind of thinking was depressing. I was fifteen years old. Life had only just begun and already I was stricken with an aching sense of disillusionment. Surely life was never meant to be like this? There had to be an answer.

CHAPTER FIFTEEN

I WAS NOT CONCENTRATING on the picture I was drawing with a crayon at OT. I'd been thinking about my adolescence and how strongly I'd felt, at fifteen, that life was never meant to be like it was. But my search for answers had led to more questions. And what now? I was scribbling trees and clouds, and birds flying over Rainbow Land, while preoccupied with pain born of the fear that I'd never be able to 'spring free'. But there *had* to be an answer.

A group of students were looking around and one of them, a red-haired, freckle-faced girl of about nineteen, went into raptures over my picture.

'Oh, isn't it good? My, aren't you clever!'

Both she and I knew a child in primary school could have done better but she called over her fellow students: 'Hey, look at this. Isn't she clever?'

They stood around me talking as if I was a precocious five-year-old.

'Oh yes, it's very good.'

'I wish I could draw like that.'

'Yes, me, too. It's absolutely marvellous.'

I said nothing, finding it easier to pretend to be too sick to respond to them in the hope that they would quickly lose interest in me. After a while, the students began talking among themselves about an ECT session they had observed.

'God, wasn't it awful! I felt sick and dizzy and I almost passed out,' a tall blonde girl said. 'My reaction really surprised me because I'm not usually squeamish.'

'Yes, it was dreadful!' someone else agreed. 'When the

patient started twitching like that, I couldn't watch.'

Suppressed anger rose in my throat as I listened to a description of how distressing it was to watch someone looking as I must have looked when my brain was tampered with in that, what now seemed to me, barbaric way. I stood up. It was time, anyway, to go back to the day hospital. Marlene and I were to have a relaxation tape session before dinner. I screwed up my childish drawing that they'd been pretending was a Picasso and dumped it in the bin.

'Oh, Jean, you missed something really good this morning,' June, the student nurse at the day hospital, said. 'We had the use of a video camera and we filmed a group of you patients sitting talking. You know how Sally keeps saying she can't make conversation? Well, we played the film back and each time it came to a part where she'd joined in, we stopped it and said to her, "Sally, you say you can't make conversation, but you're wrong. Look! There you are. Talking." She couldn't deny it because she was on film to prove it.' June turned to Nigel, the other student nurse, her eyes wide with enthusiasm. 'That's right, isn't it, Nigel? It just shows how a video camera has great potential as a therapeutic tool.'

Sally, the newest day patient, looked at me and raised her eyebrows behind their backs.

'Yes, that's what we need here,' Nigel said. 'More progressive methods.'

A therapeutic tool? Progressive methods? Why were they so bent on trying to prove there was something wrong with our perception? Wouldn't it have made more sense for them to try to understand what Sally *meant* when she kept saying she felt she could no longer make conversation?

Neither did the use of a relaxation tape make sense in the circumstances. I mean, why bother sending Marlene and me upstairs twice a week to lie on foam matting on the floor and listen to a relaxation tape? Fine, if we had a problem relaxing, but my problem was managing to keep awake. And so, too, it seemed was Marlene's.

193

'Imagine you're lying on a sunny beach ...'

The tape had only just begun and Marlene was already snoring. There was a pause somewhere during the tape where you were supposed to be in a state of deep relaxation, then, after a few minutes of silence, the 'voice' would start prattling on again about sunny beaches, against tranquil background sounds of soft, rippling water and the occasional cry of a seagull. Marlene stirred, yawned and then stood up during the silent bit and switched the tape off. She was about to go back downstairs: end of holiday.

'Er, Marlene. I don't think it's over yet,' I said.

'Oh hell!' she said. She switched it back on and lay down again. 'Wake me up when the fuckin' thing's finished.'

'I will if *I* can manage to stay awake.'

'I don't think these tapes are meant for people like us, Jean, do you? I'm forever struggling to keep alert 'cos I'm on this bloody Melleril and it knocks me out. Last thing I need is a fuckin' relaxation tape.'

'Yeah, me too,' I said. 'I could lie here and sleep all day.'

'The treatment we get at this place doesn't make sense, does it?' asked Marlene. 'I mean, when you really come to think ...'

'You're still on the sunny beach, feeling warm and comfortable and peaceful and fully relaxed ...' droned the deep, slow, male voice on the tape. 'Breathe deeply, slowly ... In. Out. In. Out. Just relax and let go of everything, let it all go...'

'When you come to think about it,' continued Marlene, 'it doesn't make any fuckin' sense.'

'Now I'm going to count to ten ...' the voice on the tape was saying gently, 'and when I get to ten, you'll open your eyes and be fully awake but you'll still be deeply relaxed. You'll still feel comfortable, peaceful and deeply, deeply relaxed. One. Two ...'

'It doesn't make sense, does it? It doesn't make any fuckin' sense at all.'

'Five. Six ...'

'No, it certainly doesn't,' I murmured sleepily.

But I suppose I did seem a nervous wreck, and not only because of the old social anxiety. I realised how shaky my hands were when I took some photographs for Mandy with her camera; each one came out blurred. And, even alongside the drowsiness, there was sometimes an intensely distressing feeling of restlessness. Years later I saw that a nurse at the day hospital had written in the Nursing Notes: 'Seems very nervous, when sitting down constantly moving arm or leg, but always very pleasant.' Mr Jordan at last told me (no one else had ever done so, as far as I can recall) that the restlessness and tremors were common side effects of the type of drugs I was taking. To lessen such effects, a drug called Kemedrin was added to my prescriptions.

In the hospital corridors one day, I stopped and leant against the wall watching life – mental institution life – pass me by. I tried to imagine the mentally sick of the Victorian era being herded through these same corridors. How many people had lived, suffered and died in this place? I'd heard it was built in the 1880s to keep about 2,500 'pauper lunatics' out of sight and mind of the public. Could their sad spirits have sunk into these walls? Sometimes, feeling an almost uncanny sensitivity to atmosphere, I thought I could sense the gloom of both past and present as if it was clinging to the walls and dripping from the ceiling.

Didn't mental patients used to be chained to the walls, doused in cold water, whirled around? What strange methods of treating people there were before the use of drugs and electric shocks. But how much progress had really been made? My thoughts turned to myself and I remembered how Mr Jordan and Dr Copeland had once pointed out that if I'd been living in an earlier period, I wouldn't have become a patient or inmate anyway. They were probably right. After all, I hadn't been talking or behaving in ways which caused concern to anybody outside the psychiatric profession. In a historical period with different ideas, I wouldn't have viewed my problems as 'medical' so would never have thought of going to my GP, asking to see a psychiatrist and agreeing to voluntary admission. There would have seemed no option but to carry on working and try to sort things out for myself. And what would have happened to me? Nothing worse than what had happened, surely? Perhaps nothing at all.

As I leant against the wall ruminating, interrupted only occasionally by one or two inmates who shuffled up asking if I'd got a cig or a light, I felt trapped. Almost as if I, too, were shackled to the wall in this awful place. I realised with dismay that I was no nearer to resolving my problems now than I had been at the age of eighteen when I'd first decided to seek psychiatric 'help'. Not only that, it seemed all I had done since then was to walk deeper and deeper into a fog from which I could find no way out.

What about my brother? I asked myself. Does one escape the conflicts of adolescence by remaining a child? But his was no easy escape. Last night he'd woken me with one of his tantrums. I'd lain in bed listening to him shouting at my parents, but what I'd really heard was an insecure child aged about five yelling, 'I hate Jean! I hate Jean! Mum wanted a girl but instead she got me. And then what happened? Four years later she got what she wanted. A girl!'

'Be quiet, Brian, you'll wake her up,' I heard Mum say.

'She's always been the favourite. I hate her!'

I didn't believe Brian really hated me. I felt he said these things because he was hurt and angry. There had been another time, not long ago, when he'd told me that I was the only person who was 'all right'. This was when he had come into my bedroom late one night and, after the usual argument about him waking me up to get to the wardrobe, we'd somehow got talking. He'd actually sat on my bed and talked about some of his insecurities and fears, and about his wish to have a girlfriend. On and on he'd talked well into the night – how much *he* had needed someone to talk to. When he left my room I sank into sleep, feeling drained but hopeful because it seemed like a breakthrough in communication with each other. The next day our relationship was back to 'normal' and it was hard to believe I hadn't only dreamt he'd sat on my bed and talked to me like that.

Although Brian spoke and acted as if he was intellectually and emotionally impaired, some things didn't seem to fit with this. For example, his knowledge and appreciation of classical music was impressive. He would, however, play his music on the record player loudly at all times of day or night. I heard Mum making sarcastic comments to him, not about his lack of consideration for others in playing the music too loudly or at inappropriate times, but about his taste in music, as if it was wrong or 'soppy' to like classical music. I wondered if Brian would have turned out quite different if he'd been brought up in a different family.

Since the onset of adolescence I had often felt angry about what I perceived to be the inappropriate and unintelligent responses of my parents, blaming them to some extent for Brian, and later perhaps me too, becoming (each in our different ways) 'screwed up'. But now I had come round to realising that my parents, like everyone else, could only behave within the bounds of their own limited capabilities or perspectives. So what was the point of being angry with them? No point in anger or blame. And nothing to rebel against any more. Not even God.

No, not even God. I remembered how a few weeks earlier I had gone to Pastor West's farewell service. He was moving to Scotland. Once again, I had heard the familiar hymn-singing, hand-clapping, gospel message, prayers. But now, even the pain and struggles and conflicts of losing my Christian beliefs had largely subsided, leaving only a dreadful emptiness, a kind of emotional deadness inside …

I was still leaning against the wall in the hospital corridor when a wild-eyed man in a long, shabby overcoat shuffled up and pestered me for a cig.

'No, I haven't got one, I don't smoke,' I said.

'Well, fuck you!' he shouted in my face. His foul breath made my stomach lurch, but since I was already leaning up against the wall I couldn't step back. I had long since stopped being afraid of these sad people, but was relieved when he went away. All the way down the corridor he shuffled along, shouting, 'Fuck you! Fuck 'em all! And fuck the whole fuckin' world!'

After the main service in the church there had been a Youth Rendezvous meeting in the hall at the back. More hand-clapping, singing and praying – along with a break for tea and biscuits. I experienced so acutely the feeling of being alone in a crowd as, with cup and saucer awkwardly balanced on my knee, I sat there dumbly, battling with the usual feelings of shyness, which now reached a peak.

I glanced round and noticed that everyone in this packed room was laughing, chatting – except for me. I don't fit in, I don't belong, I thought sadly. I don't belong anywhere. There can't be a God or surely He would help me, especially here if these are His people. Oh, why do I still keep returning to this church like a pin to a magnet?

Travelling home from church on the bus that evening I knew it was finally over, 'it' being the last bit of hope I'd cherished for so long that one day a miracle would happen that would enable me to regain my beliefs. I'd hoped that one day I'd return to church with Jackie and pick up where I'd left off when I was about sixteen, only less shy, and stronger in faith, none the worse for my worldly wanderings. Somehow, right then and there on the bus, I suddenly knew, clearer than ever before, that it could never be so. The God of my childhood and teens was not going to rise from the dead. Not now. Not ever.

Oh well, so what? People's beliefs often change as they get older, which is how it should be, I told myself. That was the last time I'd go to church and now I'd put that part of my life right behind me, and this time I really would let go. I'd stop looking back. Even so, it had been a lovely dream while it lasted.

It had started to rain; the bus window was so splattered with raindrops that I could hardly see through it, but there was another reason for my blurred vision. I paid my fare hardly daring to turn properly and then I returned my gaze to the window. Don't cry, Jean. For heaven's sake, don't cry. This was so unlike me. I rarely cried at all these days and certainly not in front of people. I surely wouldn't cry here in front of a whole busload of people.

I fought tremendously hard to hold back my tears but they just seeped out of my eyes like water from a leaking tap. Soon my face was hot, my nose running and my cheeks wet with scalding tears. But at least they were silent tears. With my face still riveted to the window, nobody could see me, nobody need know, although as the grey terraced houses, the parade of shops, the cinema on the corner, sped by through a blur of rain and tears, I was becoming increasingly worried about getting off. Opting for a swift solution, I stumbled down the aisle, my long hair hiding my face, and got off a few stops earlier than usual.

Walking through the cold wind and rain, my face stinging as my tears flowed unchecked to mingle with the elements, I realised, through a throbbing sensation from within, that at least I felt more alive when I cried. It was worse not to be able to cry. And to feel dead inside was the worst feeling of all …

'Fuck you! Fuck you! Fuck you!'

The reappearance of the 'Fuck you!' man returned me to the bleak hospital corridor. When he reached me he shuffled to a halt and stopped swearing. I was about to tell him again that, no, I hadn't got a cig, but this time he didn't ask. He stared intently at my face.

'You're crying,' he said.

I pressed my hands against my wet cheeks. He was right.

LOOKING BACK 9

I WAS FIFTEEN WHEN I went with Dad to a meeting at the Pentecostal church he used to go to in his teens. I was struck by how happy and uninhibited everyone seemed, with a spontaneity similar to that I could remember from Salvation Army meetings: people shouting 'Yes, Lord. Amen!' 'Hallelujah!' 'Praise Him!' and clapping their hands to the joyful choruses.

A teenage boy came out to the front and gave his 'testimony'. He spoke about his life and how he had become a 'born again' Christian. How different he was from the boys I knew. He seemed to have found a real meaning and purpose to life, and I longed to be the same.

All noise in the packed church subsided while a small man with a loud voice proclaimed the 'Good News', that old, familiar story of Jesus Christ, Son of God, coming to earth to die on the cross and rising up from the dead so that 'whosoever believeth in Him should not perish but have everlasting life'.

As I sat and listened to the Gospel, an old flame was rekindled within me. Would it be possible for me to regain something of that strong, simple faith I'd had in early childhood? Could the meaning and message of the gospel have any relevance for me personally in my day-to-day living?

It was time now for the 'appeal'. Those who felt the call to commit their lives to Christ were invited to kneel at the front as a public declaration that they were asking Jesus to come into their heart. This 'accepting Jesus', which could be done either publicly or privately, was what was meant by being 'saved' or 'born again'. My father made his way to the front, and knelt in tears.

I went home with the Gospel Message buzzing around inside my head. Something about that church got hold of me right from the start. It was like a powerful magnet pulling me to it.

I persuaded Jackie to come with me and we started going regularly. Someone gave us a tract about being 'born again'. We took it into the Cellar Bar one night and, there in the dim lights and din, we read and reread it, discussing each part, hardly hearing the pop songs blasting out from the jukebox.

I spent restless months lingering in a kind of limbo, buffeted by doubts, but feeling a strong urge to commit myself. I thought I couldn't be 'saved' until I could believe without doubts, since faith was obviously essential to salvation – 'whosoever believeth'. Then, while I was lying awake one night, I realised something.

That's it! I thought excitedly. I don't have to wait until these conflicts and doubts go. I can come 'just as I am'. I got out of bed, knelt at the side, and gave myself to Him who understands our innermost thoughts and feelings.

After that night, I tried hard to be a good Christian. I prayed daily, read my Bible and sought God's guidance in every aspect of my life. I was young, idealistic and very sincere.

After Dad returned to church I think he did try to curb his bad moods, but during yet another period of family squabbles, sulks and disruption, he told me he was looking for other accommodation. He said again I would have to hurry up and decide whom I wanted to live with – 'her or me'. But I knew now that I needn't make that decision because soon I'd be old enough to leave home. Roll on sixteen.

By the time my sixteenth birthday came, my parents were still living together, and religion had become as much a part of my life as breathing. Stretched taut with spiritual yearning, I sought the fullness of God.

My soul thirsteth for thee, my flesh longeth
for thee in a dry and thirsty land, where no
water is.(Psalm 63:1)

But questions, questions, questions, kept springing, unwanted
and unbidden, to my mind. What did this mean? What did that
mean? How could I know for certain that the Bible was true?
And supposing I had got it all wrong. I mean, supposing that
God didn't even exist? My mind was forever demanding
answers, throwing up doubts, engaging in an intense
intellectual and emotional struggle to understand, to believe, to
know. I tried hard to blot the doubts from my mind, hold my
critical faculties in abeyance and accept Him by faith as I
buried myself more and more in a world of bibles, hymns and
prayers.

I struggled over difficult theological concepts, prayed hard
for spiritual enlightenment, strength and guidance ... and I fell
down before the resurrected Christ, saying like the father in the
Bible story: 'Lord, I believe; help thou mine unbelief.'

Again, I felt the strength of that bond between Dad and me.
We looked to our beliefs, hoping to invoke the power of God to
smooth out our family problems. We wanted miracles. And why
not? For did not Jesus Himself say that when two or more
people were gathered together in His name, He would be right
there in the midst of them? So together, just the two of us, we
got down on our knees in my bedroom and prayed each in turn
out loud, self-consciously at first, then more boldly as
inhibitions and defences dropped.

How can I describe those sweet moments I spent together
with my earthly father and my Heavenly Father, bound by
cords of love, both human and divine? The sense of wonder
and awe which filled my heart as we knelt before the throne of
God defies description.

At least that's the way it felt at the time. But feelings,
especially intense adolescent feelings, cannot be trusted. Of
course, I know better now, having learnt such a lot since then.
And yet, it's as if a small part of me was left behind in the past.

It's still there now, wandering through the graveyard of lost beliefs searching for I know not what.

CHAPTER SIXTEEN

EVERY MORNING I PASSED a bench in the grounds where a man sat dejectedly, body slumped forward, head down low. I could imagine his picture on a poster with a caption urging people to give generously for the mentally ill. Although not restrained in a building as past inmates had been, he seemed doomed to exist inside the prison of himself, forlorn and hopeless; one of society's misfits.

My mind barely registered seeing him until the day he wasn't there. Each morning after that, the empty bench reminded me of this man. Perhaps I should have attempted some small caring gesture, at least tried saying 'Good morning' to him. And now it was too late.

But it wasn't too late for me to give Arnold a cup of coffee. Arnold, a day patient, was a stroke victim. The staff didn't make him join in the therapy like the other patients as he didn't seem capable, so he was left to sit and vegetate most of the time. Occasionally, a nurse, perhaps trying to be cruel to be kind, snapped at him to 'Get a grip on yourself, Arnold!' He used to be able to get a grip; he used to be a senior police officer. But now he was 'unfit for duties' as he could hardly walk or talk, couldn't use his hands properly and dribbled down his chin.

At breaks Caroline would wheel in the trolley and leave cups and two big jugs of coffee on a table in the middle of the room for us to pour. I noticed Arnold sitting there one day while the rest of us drank coffee. I waited for someone else to notice, but nobody did. 'OK, Jean, you rotten coward. You *can't* get out of this one,' I said to myself. I was shaking inside as I stood up. I don't think it would have been a problem if there had been just the two of us, but I was self-conscious about walking over and speaking to him in front of a room full of watching people.

'Arnold, do you take sugar?' I asked, wondering if he could understand and reply.

He nodded, and mouthed the words, 'Two please' holding up two fingers. After that it was easy to get Arnold's coffee every day, and the way he always managed to stutter out a 'Thank you', which later became, 'Thank you, Jean', was deeply moving.

Mr Jordan rescued me from some of my attendances at the OT building by arranging for me to help in the library a few afternoons a week. The library was in the main hospital block, somewhere down those dismal corridors.

Mr Jordan introduced me to Hazel, the librarian, a slender, fair-haired, attractive young woman. She asked me which books I liked. I didn't read much now but had recently started rereading a book about Helen Keller. I'd always been interested in how people overcame various kinds of difficulties in communicating.

'I'm reading a book about Helen Keller,' I replied.

'Hell and what?' Mr Jordan asked.

'Helen Keller.'

'Hell and what?'

'She said Helen Keller,' Hazel explained, smiling. 'You know, the deaf and blind woman.'

The library consisted of a large room with shelves all round and some chairs. It had the appearance, if not quite the same atmosphere, of any local library. The main difference was that the chairs were often used by long-stay patients who sat staring into space and muttering to themselves instead of reading. To the left of this main room was a separate smaller locked room, a staff library. Occasionally I was given some books to replace on the shelves in there and found it contained interesting looking books. Hazel once caught me engrossed in the pages of *The Case of Mary Bell* and reminded me that these books were not for patients.

A white-coated male nurse came into the library one day with a few docile-looking patients.

'They're from a locked ward,' Hazel informed me. 'I'll introduce you to Toby. He's really cute.'

She called one of the patients over; a small ginger-haired man whose face was covered in pimples. Like the others, he seemed heavily sedated.

'Toby, this is Jean,' Hazel said.

He held out his hand to me. 'Hello, Jean,' he drawled. 'I'm very pleased to meet you.'

'Toby can sing,' Hazel said brightly. 'Toby, show Jean what you can do. Sing your song for her.'

He looked at me, blushed, and stared down at the floor. 'Aw, no,' he said coyly.

'Oh come on, Toby, please,' Hazel said.

After some more persuasion, he sang to the 'Happy Birthday' tune:

> Largactil for me
> Largactil for me
> I do like Largactil
> Largactil for me.

I smiled and clapped the circus show along with the others, but my guts were gripped by the same uneasy feeling I'd had at the day hospital when a nurse had cajoled an embarrassed Betsy into jumping about saying: 'I am silly. I am silly ...'

One of the patients who came often to sit in the library was Samuel, a short man with greying hair, who wore a shabby jacket with a dark-red bow tie. He would sit quietly, and then suddenly spring to his feet, shouting: 'I hate the Nazis! I hate the Nazis! They killed my mother and my father and my sister.'

After his outburst he would return to brooding, before starting up again. 'They say this is a hospital and they tell me I'm here because I am mentally disturbed. What does this "mentally disturbed" mean? I try to understand what happened to me and to my family. I ask myself why? WHY? It was sadistic, brutal torture and murder. They murdered my dear mother and father, my gentle sister. I hate the Nazis! I hate them!' His voice, slow and deliberate at first, grew louder and angrier, his face contorted in the anguish of remembering, then he slumped back into his seat and lapsed again into silence.

One thing soothed Samuel's troubled mind: Tchaikovsky's *Swan Lake*. Every few weeks Hazel held a 'Records Hour' in the library. At the sound of *Swan Lake* Samuel's troubled expression was transformed into one of serenity. He would lean back with closed eyes, humming the tune and smiling contentedly as if the music had the power to transport him far away from High Royds, and further back than the horrors of the Nazi regime. Back, back, gently back to a happy, peaceful time that had been preserved somewhere among the dust and debris in his brain like a flower in the desert.

One day during the Records Hour, Samuel came in when I was playing a Supremes record. His usual tortured expression wrung my heart and, hoping to help ease his pain, I searched among the pile of records for his beloved *Swan Lake*. But too late. He stood still for a moment, listening to the Tamla Motown disco sound of 'Baby Love'. Then he threw up his arms in disgust and stormed out with an angry shout: 'RUBBISH!'

One of the perks of working in the library was Horace. Horace was a library helper from a long-stay ward. Before his admission he had been a tramp, sleeping rough, stealing food and clothing. It might have been easier for him as a young man but, having reached his sixties with health failing, it was a tough life, devoid of the basic comforts most people take for granted. He kept appearing before the courts for stealing and when the judge sentenced him to prison, which to Horace meant food and shelter, he would say gratefully, 'Oh, thank you very much, sir. That's most kind of you.'

Finally, he was sent to High Royds, which had become his home. When there was talk of getting long-stay patients back into the community, poor old Horace was extremely worried that he might be discharged.

Horace was a great storyteller. He kept Hazel and me amused by telling us interesting stories about his life on the streets. He told of his escapades in later years of trying to get himself sent to prison, such as how one night he broke into a food factory, turned on the lights and helped himself to a pork pie. He was most indignant that the policeman who came to arrest him wouldn't allow him to finish his pie before taking him to the cells.

Horace's tales, like all life stories, probably contained a mixture of fact and fiction. He had the gift of telling his sometimes sad but mostly funny stories in a way that made them sparkle with life. Many times I sat with him while he rolled cigarettes or smoked Woodbines and recounted another instalment from the Life of Horace. He could make me laugh, no matter how tired and low I was feeling. Many of the staff, even, had a soft spot for this friendly, likeable, apparently simple chap who, behind their backs, could imitate them perfectly, demonstrating a shrewd perception of their little idiosyncrasies.

'Guess who this is,' he would say to Hazel and me, then he would take off several of the doctors in turn, getting the voice and mannerisms of each one just right as he enacted a little scene.

Each week Horace did the 'ward rounds', taking a trolley of books to the back wards, including some locked wards. Hazel suggested I accompany him. The first time I went with him there was a commotion in the corridors. A few male patients stampeded through with male nurses in close pursuit. Horace and I, who'd been wheeling the book trolley along the corridor, got caught up in this and, afterwards, I found myself alone up against the wall where I'd been shoved while people raced past. Horace had run off at the first sign of trouble, abandoning the trolley and me. I found him waiting for me further along the corridor.

'Horace! You're not looking after me properly,' I teased him playfully.

After that, whenever we went on the ward rounds together, he assigned himself the role of my protector and proudly told Hazel and other staff members that he was looking after me.

I soon became aware that Thornville was not like some of the other wards. The back wards we visited, pushing the library trolley, were grim, overcrowded places, reeking of piss and shit, with beds sandwiched together. There were no pale, rosebud Ophelias among whiskery-faced women who dribbled and grimaced and spat. Trying to find romantic literary depictions of madness here would be as futile as trying to ride a rainbow or dance on clouds while the sky spewed out black, bitter rain over all that moved.

A few lost-looking souls shuffled around the area in front of the rows of beds where we stood with the trolley. The others, old, deformed, shrivelled, were sitting or lying on rubber-sheeted mattresses in a prison of beds. Belsen-thin. Sunken eyes. Rocking. Chewing. Saliva dribbling down their chins. Rattling the bed ends, beating their chests, tugging at clumps of hair, while snake-like tongues occasionally darted in and out of their mouths. I looked closer. No, they were not all the same. There were noisy patients, who reminded me of my brother in the way they banged, tapped, and made animal sounds, and quiet patients, with stone-fixed expressions. A mixed bag of misery.

Did the white-coated workers barricade emotions daily to separate and safeguard their minds from those who made up this overspill of drab decay? But I was unschooled and unshielded, still young enough to see and feel it all with open-hearted anguish.

To enter the locked wards, we had to ring the bell to summon the attendant whose eye would appear at the peephole. After stating our business, we waited, listening to the sounds of unlocking and unbolting. As soon as we entered, the heavy door was firmly closed, the large bolts drawn, the key turned. A chill feeling gripped my stomach. I was locked inside ...

The first time I went into a locked ward, I followed the burly attendant apprehensively down the short, inner corridor to the main room. The keys that hung from his belt jangled as he walked. I wondered what to expect, but most of the patients in this male ward looked so heavily sedated that it was hard to appreciate the need for the lock or, for that matter, for the books we were bringing.

Yet, in all the sad, drab, pee-smelling wards we went into with the books, there was always someone, perhaps only one patient out of the whole ward, who still possessed the faculties and motivation to read. In one of the locked wards, Nancy, a small woman with big dark eyes and sparrow-like arms and legs, rushed to greet us each week and chatted to me excitedly about the books she'd read, before looking along the rows of books on the trolley to choose some more. Why was this woman being buried alive in here? I looked around at her companions to see whom she might converse with, but some were cabbage-like and silent, others were weeping and wailing and gnashing their teeth.

How could anyone who had a mind sharp enough to think and reason survive in this bleak environment? Was it too much to hope that these books Nancy rushed for so eagerly each week were a lifeline for her? Could they help prevent soul-death? Even in this hell?

In a male locked ward a man in a similar position to Nancy had apparently found a different aid to survival, something to alleviate the boredom of the day if new, naïve visitors came. His name was Victor and the first time I met him, he came up to me, smiling, with his arm outstretched wanting me to 'shake hands'.

'I wouldn't if I were you,' a tired-looking male nurse warned me, but Victor was a small, thin man and I couldn't see any harm in it, so I allowed him to grasp my hand.

The handshake didn't stop at the normal stage. Still retaining his oh-so-polite pleased-to-meet-you smile, he squeezed my hand in an iron grip until I yelled in pain and the nurse, whom I now wished I'd heeded, managed to yank him away from me.

LOOKING BACK 10

I WAS NEARING MY seventeenth birthday when it became impossible for me to continue being a Christian. Questions and doubts had long been rocking the boat but what finally capsized me was to do with the Christian doctrine about hell. Accept Jesus as Saviour or be damned for eternity? No peace of mind for ever and ever? Surely nobody deserved that? Many people on earth were suffering enough and if God wouldn't at least grant them relief in death, then what kind of a God was I supposed to be believing in? Of course, I had to reject the 'sweetness' of my religion along with the 'cruelty'. Things couldn't be 'true' or 'not true' just because that's how I wanted them to be. I had to let go.

But how could I let go of Him who meant everything to me and replace Him with – nothing? I read my favourite, beautiful hymns once more. Wanting, needing, to believe so much, the hymn book's clear, black print dissolved into a blur of tears.

A grey cloud descended over me. As a result of my belief system breaking down, I was suffering the devastating loss of ultimate meaning. What point was there in anything? Why bother to breathe? In bed I gazed up at the sky through the gap in my curtains, and wept and tossed about feverishly, gripped by a sense of misdirected energy. It seemed that life was a maze leading to dead ends no matter what routes we chose. Did we have any choices anyway? How could Christians reconcile free will with predestination? Wasn't Judas's fate mapped out for him long before he was born?

My thoughts went shooting off freely down unexplored avenues, having been unleashed from the basic assumptions on

211

which my sense of 'reality' had been founded. God? Heaven and hell? Eternal suffering? Good/Evil? Right/Wrong? The old 'black/white' world of childhood collapsed. I was confused with so many different ideas, many of them nihilistic. No God? No free will? No ultimate meaning? These ideas can be difficult to assimilate amidst the turmoil of being 'sixteen, going on seventeen'.

My old questions about right and wrong turned into: on what values or basic assumptions should we base our morality? If I couldn't sort that one out, how could I have any opinions or know what decisions to make in the day-to-day issues which confronted me? And how could I sort out my views on matters like abortion, euthanasia, pacifism, politics, capital punishment and so on, if I didn't even know on what to base my views?

The concept of 'I' and 'me' provided me with more than enough food for thought to choke upon. WHAT AM I?– the Jackpot Question – became of central importance. I felt desperately alone, fearing that no one else on earth had ever wondered what a human being is.

It wasn't just that this teenage religious thing had soured. No, my grief over lost beliefs went deeper than that. All my life Jesus had been the Friend who was always there. Admittedly, I'd had strong religious doubts around the age of twelve when I left the Salvation Army. But I'd never lost Him completely before. Not like this. How was I to make sense, alone, of this world around me, which I was so painfully dissatisfied with?

The 'new me' emerged. Jean the Christian became Jean the Rebel. I wore shorter skirts, heavy eye-liner and was drinking, smoking and swearing like the rest of them. Caught up on a merry-go-round of a social whirl, I was out every night at pubs, nightclubs and discos, often until the early hours of the morning. I kept my conflicts and confusion about religion and life to myself. Nobody must know I was not the modern, carefree teenager I was pretending to be.

I remained hung up about questions of right and wrong.

When kissing and petting, as I frequently did with boys I neither knew nor liked, I felt I was not acting in accordance with my true feelings. I needed to be me but I needed to belong. So I kept trying to pull the two opposing needs together into some kind of uneasy compromise. I did keep my virginity though, still saving it for the 'right' boyfriend, if such a person existed. Boyfriends could go so far but no further. Definitely no further.

I tried to weather the violence and misery around me with a cynical and detached 'Well, that's life' attitude. I never even thought of going to the police when I was set upon and badly beaten up one night. Or when, on another night, while walking home alone in the dark (I wondered if it was my fault for doing that), a beer-smelling man dragged me on to some waste ground. He pinned me flat on my back in the mud and gravel, his strong animal-hungry body heavy on top of me. Was it at some time during the lengthy and sickening sexual assault he subjected me to that a part of me finally accepted that life was just a load of shit piled up on top of shit? I told Mum about the sex attack but she didn't seem interested. That hurt. I told Dad and he said if this had happened I must have 'asked for it'. That hurt even more.

Teenage life seemed so gut-achingly depressing. Of the old friends I knew from way back at junior school, Shirley had an abortion at fifteen and Sylvia joined a cult at sixteen. A previous boyfriend, Barry, committed suicide at seventeen ...

And the drugs scene saddened me. I went to the Tempest Folk Club a few times with Phil who was a nice lad when he wasn't too stoned on acid or snow. Leaning against Phil's shoulder, the words of one of my favourite Bob Dylan songs, 'Mr Tambourine Man', mingled with the woozy thoughts in my head.

Through an alcohol haze I grieved for lost innocence, while thinking: Hey, Mr Tambourine Man, I know now that you're a heroin dealer.

I learnt to type at night school and left my job at the factory for

*a typing job at Lee's, an electrical wholesalers. It was less
boring than the assembly line – but not much. Mandy, my old
friend from Rossfields, worked at a shoe shop near Lee's and
we began meeting at lunchtime each day. We soon got to know
each other much better than when we were schoolgirls and our
friendship grew strong. At that time Mandy seemed more
'innocent' than me and my other friends. This appealed to me,
perhaps because I kept wishing I could regain some of the
innocence I felt I'd lost.*

*I was seventeen when Steve became my steady boyfriend.
Good-looking and sexy, he could have had his pick of
girlfriends, but he asked me to dance at a disco and soon we
were 'together'.*

*The psychedelic lighting in the Stardust illuminated my
white cardigan and Steve's shirt in contrast to the surrounding
dimness. Feeling groggy with beer but more drunk on the
surreal atmosphere of the place, I listened, dreamily, to the
haunting sound of Procol Harum's 'A Whiter Shade of Pale'.*

Then suddenly – puff!

*The music stopped; the room was flooded with harsh, bright
light revealing chipped tables, tatty wall décor, a dirty floor.
'Time, please!' Handsome princes were transformed back to
pimpled-faced, bleary-eyed frogs sitting at tables littered with
half-finished glasses of beer, cigarette packets, puddles on
beer-mats and ugly over-stuffed ashtrays. Screwed-up eyes
soon became accustomed to the light, ears to the silence of
stopped music as our senses quickly adjusted to the way the
scene had changed in an instant. But somewhere in that
disorientating instant, in the tiny gap between the breaking of
one illusion and the adjusting to another, there flashed a
moment of truth – or a moment of madness: call it what you
will. A glimpse into the reality of our unrealities – or was it the
unreality of our realities? Did others experience that, too, or
was it just me? I shivered.*

*It's all an illusion, I thought, as I gulped down the remains
of my lager while Adam, the friendly barman, stood at my table*

214

waiting for my empty glass. Life's one big illusion that we create out of the whole fabric of illusions we're immersed in from birth to death. And for what purpose?

*   'Hi, Jean. Do you know any good jokes?' Adam asked with a grin.*

CASE NO. 10826

Recent Progress:
(1) For a year she has attended the Day Hospital regularly and has always been a good time-keeper.

(2) She is always neatly-dressed.

(3) She co-operates in two schemes of group therapy and is able to write with real skill and enthusiasm, having a good command of English. There is every indication that she was able to achieve a high standard at school. Recently her own activities at the Day Hospital have been extended, so that she is working in the library on four half days per week, where she is interested and always helpful to the librarian.

(4) She also spends two half-days with Mrs Green's department, one session for typing and one session for the art class.

Proposals:
One is left with the impression that she might benefit from Modecate injections and perhaps a course of E.C.T.

Dr Shaw

CHAPTER SEVENTEEN

'DID YOU KNOW YOUR mother's having an affair?'

Mandy and I were lying in bed one Sunday morning, having spent the night at her cousin Sarah's house.

'What makes you think that?'

'Your mother told me so herself,' Mandy replied, pulling herself up into a sitting position and, inadvertently, robbing me of my share of covers. 'Remember I told you I saw her last week at the bus stop when I was going to my grandma's? Well, she just started telling me. I was dead embarrassed. Did you know about it?'

I shivered, retrieved some of the pink quilted bedspread and curled up into a ball. 'Yeah. I know.'

'Does it bother you?'

'I don't like to see Dad getting hurt, but I suppose if Mum wants to have an affair, it's her business.'

As I was saying this, Sarah, a young divorcee, was coming into the bedroom with a tray of coffee.

'What? Your mam's having an affair?' Sarah exclaimed. 'That's awful!' She stood in the doorway in a white frilly nightgown, her corn-gold hair wound up in large, spiky pink rollers.

'So what? Lots of people have affairs,' I pointed out.

'Yes, I know, but you don't expect that sort of thing of your parents, do you?' Sarah said, sitting on the bed with the tray.

'Why not? Parents are ordinary, fallible people, too,' I commented, stirring my coffee.

But a dangerous game was being played out. More so than I knew at the time. Years later, Dad told me how he'd gone out in search of Roy with a carving knife hidden beneath his coat (fortunately, he didn't find him that night). 'Did you really intend to kill him?' I asked. His reply: 'I just wanted to spoil his good looks.'

Anger towards my mother bubbled up inside me. I waited until I was alone with her. She was sitting on the settee reading the *Daily Mirror*. I sat down beside her.

'Mum, why did you tell Mandy that you're carrying on with Roy?'

She looked up from the paper. 'Tell Mandy?' she asked with a vacant look in her eyes.

'Don't pretend you don't know what I'm talking about. Mandy said you saw her at the bus stop last week and you told her.'

'Well, yeah, I did. It doesn't matter.' She went back to reading the paper.

'It matters to me, and you embarrassed Mandy as well.'

'Mandy? I don't see why. She's old enough to know about these things.'

I gave up and turned on the TV. She didn't seem to have any idea what the problem was.

Later that evening she turned to me and said, 'I think Roy's coming for Christmas.'

'What?' I thought I'd got beyond being surprised by things that went on in our family. But this made me sit up and listen. 'You've invited him here? To our house?'

'Yes,' she said. Her eyes were shining.

'What about Dad?'

She shrugged her shoulders.

'You can't be serious,' I said, but the look on her face told me she saw nothing wrong or problematic about inviting her 28-year-old lover to spend Christmas with us. Nothing at all.

Things came to a head with my parents one day when, after a squabble, Mum announced tearfully that she was leaving.

'Don't come back!' Dad shouted after her. 'You stupid old bag!'

'Come inside, Dad. Just let her go,' I said, putting my hand on his shoulder, but he hadn't finished yet.

'You whore!' he shouted, before slamming the door and locking it. He turned to me. 'She's nowt but a friggin' whore. Any love I once had for her has been killed.'

'Sit down, Dad. I'll put the kettle on.'

'I'm not sorry she's gone. I'm better off without her.'

'Do you want tea or coffee?'

'She's a scrubber!'

'Or hot chocolate?'

'If she wants to come back I won't let her in. I'll get the locks changed tomorrow.'

Next day when it was time to set off for the day hospital, I was reluctant to leave Dad alone in his distressed state.

'You could ring Mr Jordan and tell him my mum's left home and I'm too upset to go to the hospital today,' I suggested.

This backfired. Mr Jordan advised Dad to accompany me to the hospital.

When we arrived, Mr Jordan had arranged for Dr Copeland to see me. My father waited downstairs while I went into the office with Dr Copeland and Mr Jordan. After discussing what had happened, Dr Copeland said, 'You're coping well with the situation. I can see there's no need for me to arrange your admission.'

'What? Of course I don't need to be admitted!' I said, alarmed at the thought.

Dr Copeland and Mr Jordan exchanged glances and smiled. 'Well, now that we've seen you we know you're all right, but your father said on the phone that you were very upset.'

'Yes, I know, but I'm nowhere near upset enough to need hospitalising,' I said quickly.

The phone rang for Dr Copeland and he left in a hurry. I went downstairs to the sitting room, and Mr Jordan took my father into the office. When Dad came out, he'd obviously been crying. Mr Jordan spoke to me while Dad waited downstairs.

'Jean, I'm concerned about your father. I mean, when a man

breaks down and cries like that, something's wrong, isn't it?'

'Is it?' I asked. I'd often seen Dad cry.

'Do you ever feel like hitting your mother? If I were your dad I'd have thumped her by now.'

'Would you? Oh well, I'm sure wife-battering is a mature, sensible response,' I said sarcastically. I wondered if he'd said this to test my reaction. The staff often said things I couldn't believe they really meant, so I could only conclude it must be to see how patients reacted to what they said.

'It would serve her right. I wouldn't have allowed her to humiliate me all this time,' Mr Jordan said.

'It's not fair of you to judge her when you've only heard one side of the story,' I pointed out.

'Well, has she really been talking about having her lover stay for Christmas? With your father there as well? That's ludicrous.'

'Yes, but perhaps she didn't know how this hurt him.'

'Oh, come off it, Jean. How could she not know?'

I thought maybe my parents were childlike and naïve rather than vindictive, though I couldn't try to explain that without it seeming as if I was the one who was childlike and naïve.

'Your father needs you a lot,' Mr Jordan said.

'I know.'

'He needs you more than you need him.'

'I don't know about that, but I do sometimes think … well, it often seems as if …' I stopped. How much should I say? What about loyalty to my family? Was I being fair?

'Yes, go on,' Mr Jordan urged me.

'Dad's always leant on me, cried on my shoulder, confided in me about adult things even when I was a kid. It's almost as if I were the parent and he was the child. He often tells me his troubles and asks for my advice.'

'Do you think that's good or bad for you?'

'For me? Maybe a bit of both,' I said, thinking of how it at least might have redressed the balance a bit of being treated as a psychiatric patient with no valid views. Two extremes cancelling each other out perhaps? 'But to be honest,' I continued, 'I'm more worried now about my dependency on my parents than *their* dependency on me. I don't know how I'd cope, either financially, practically or emotionally, without them.'

'You *could* manage, Jean,' Mr Jordan said reassuringly. 'Your lack of confidence doesn't surprise me, but you're far more capable of coping than you think.'

After tea that evening Dad called me to the window. I saw a dejected figure sitting on the garden wall, with coat collar up, head bent, shoulders hunched up against the wind.

Dad opened the window and started to shout: 'Why don't you go to him now? Won't he have you?' But he turned and whispered to me, 'What shall I do, Jean? Tell me what to do.'

'Let her come in, Dad,' I begged.

'No, I won't,' he said, but after a pause, he called out to her: 'If you want to come in for tonight you can do, you silly bitch.'

At first she didn't move.

'Either you come in right now or I'll lock you out again.'

Slowly she walked inside, tears streaming down her face.

This must have heralded the end of the affair. From then on there was no more talk of Roy coming for Christmas, no more did she talk to Mandy about the affair, no more jumping each time the telephone rang, no more whispering and giggling into the phone. And no more sparkle in her dull, lifeless eyes.

Mum said she'd walked the streets, enquired at a hotel but found it much too expensive, and spent the night on some wasteland.

'The woman's mentally ill,' Dad said to me. 'Tell me, Jean, would anyone in their right mind go off and sleep in a field like that?'

'Maybe they would if they were very unhappy,' I said.

I'd thought my mother and I were so different – I even used to wonder if she'd been given the wrong baby by mistake in the hospital when I was born. But were we *really* so different? I'd be unhappy with a life like hers. Perhaps she was, too.

'Mum, why did you work in the mill at fourteen?' I asked

when just the two of us were together. 'Didn't you want something more?'

'I'd no choice 'cos me wage was needed. I won a scholarship to go to grammar school but I couldn't go 'cos we needed money.'

She must have had academic ability, I thought with admiration. Not many children from our kind of background won scholarships.

'Do you have regrets?'

'No, there'd be no point, would there? I mean you just do what you have to do. Nobody needs to know the stuff they teach you at school anyhow. But it was sad for me brother. Now he's the one who must have regrets. He was only sixteen when he had to get married and do whatever jobs he could to support his wife and kiddie. It's a real shame because he was right clever at school and he could've gone far, being a boy.'

I lay in bed that night thinking of wasted lives. But why should Mum's brother have gone far 'being a boy'? What about girls? What about the needs, aspirations and abilities of women?

'We'd like you to go to the psychology department to do some tests,' Mr Jordan informed me one morning.

I hadn't known there was a psychology department at High Royds. A morning spent there proved to be more interesting than OT. A petite young woman with long auburn hair shook my hand and introduced herself as Laura Barnes, a clinical psychologist. She showed me pictures and told me to make up a story around them, gave me a list of things which people might fear, such as flying, spiders, having a serious operation, and told me to tick along a continuum ranging from 'no fear at all' to 'a very strong fear', and she gave me sentence beginnings to finish off. Finally, there was the IQ test, which involved choosing which numbers and shapes fitted into a pattern sequence and so on. The intelligence test started off being very easy and became progressively harder but, not wanting to appear dim, I forced my sleepy, rusty brain to creak into action as it hadn't done in ages. All tests finished, I thought no more about them until Dr Copeland and Mr Jordan called me into the top-floor office at the day hospital a few days later.

'I've found out we have someone here at the day hospital who has an IQ that is well above average,' Dr Copeland said, smiling. 'That's what your test result shows.'

'Does it?' I said, with only mild interest. I did not believe that tests which measured an aptitude for solving pencil and paper puzzles could ever tap the kind of intelligence linked to the qualities of character that *really* mattered.

'Tell me why you're a patient,' Dr Copeland said.

'Because I'm mentally ill,' I replied, deciding to face up to that head on.

'Is that what you want me to believe?'

'Well, I am, aren't I?'

'In my opinion, no,' he said.

He leafed back through the pages of my case notes, reading them quietly for a while.

'OK,' he said, 'so you became confused about religion and got hung up on questioning what life's all about. Sounds to me like the normal turmoils of an intelligent adolescent, though no doubt intensified in your case by your home life.'

Intensified, too, by my experiences in Thornville, I thought bitterly.

'I'm not an adolescent now,' I reminded him, 'and I'm still as confused as ever about religion, and life in general.'

'So what? So are lots of people,' he said. 'Christ, I often wonder what life's all about.'

He paused, lit a cigarette, and stared at me till I felt uncomfortable.

'You haven't yet convinced me that you are, or were, in any way sick, though for some reason you believe that you are,' he said. 'It's clear to Dave Jordan and me that you're as different from the other patients here as chalk from cheese. I can find in you absolutely no trace of mental illness.'

He inhaled on his cigarette, held his head back and breathed

223

out slowly. 'Stop seeing yourself as mentally ill, Jean.'

I stared at Dr Copeland in amazement. It had taken me some time to get used to the idea that I was mentally ill, and now he was talking like this. But he was a psychiatrist so he, more than most people, must have known very well where I'd been taught to perceive myself as sick.

'You're not supposed to say that, are you?' I said mischievously. 'Shouldn't you be calling me a good girl for admitting that I'm mentally ill? Don't I get brownie points or something for showing "insight"?'

'I don't think this is something you should be joking about.'

I stopped laughing at once. 'OK. Why was I given ECT?'

'I can't speak for other doctors. I wouldn't prescribe ECT for you.'

'Well, if you don't think I'm sick, why prescribe drugs?'

For the first time he looked uncomfortable. 'That's ... that's difficult to explain,' he said, rubbing his forehead. 'You've been on drugs for a long time and I personally would like to take you off them but ...'

'But what? Does Dr Shaw ...'

'Have you ever thought of leaving home?' he asked, changing the subject.

'Yes, but I'm hardly in a position to do that now, am I? I threw that opportunity away when I chucked up me last job. It was the middle of the afternoon and I felt so tired and bored that I couldn't stand it any more. I just grabbed me coat and went home.'

'I'd have probably done the same in your situation. I don't know how people can stick boring jobs. For instance, I often wonder how people can, say, work on a factory assembly line. I wouldn't be able to stand that for one single day.'

'Really?' A tiny chink of light penetrated my blindfold. Maybe it wasn't me after all? Still, something scared me about the way he was talking. 'You'll think I'm sick if I tell you what I did one night,' I said. 'Roy, Mum's fancy man, rang and she got dressed up like a teenager and rushed out to meet him. Call me I'll come running! I think I wanted her to worry about me.

Anyway, I took off and stayed out all night. Slept in a bus parked up in a depot. That's a sick thing to do, isn't it?'

'In your circumstances, I think not.'

I eyed Dr Copeland curiously. It was a refreshing change to listen to a psychiatrist who was refusing to find 'symptoms' in everything. He stubbed out his cigarette, looked at me and sighed.

'What can I say to you? A shuffle of social factors and you could be sitting here behind this desk doing my job. You're easily as intelligent as I am.'

'You've a lot of faith in IQ tests but I'm enjoying the flattery,' I said, smiling.

'No, you're wrong there. I haven't drawn my conclusions only from an IQ test,' he said. 'I've had conversations with you on a wide range of topics, including religion and philosophy. With no disrespect to the other patients downstairs, I couldn't discuss things on that level with any of them. And I can't find anything wrong with you.'

'Don't you think I'm depressed?' I asked.

'Well, you don't report any symptoms, such as early-morning wakening, which fits with a clinical depression,' he replied.

'No, I don't wake early,' I agreed, wondering how anyone could wake early when on such knock-out drugs, 'but I'm so dissatisfied with life. Sometimes I feel such ... despair.'

'Dissatisfied, sad, downhearted, yes, OK, but that's not mental illness.' Dr Copeland leaned forward and spoke with a tone of urgency. 'For heaven's sake, Jean, do *something* with your abilities. Don't just throw them away. It's such a terrible waste.'

LOOKING BACK 11

IN THE EARLY SUMMER of 1968 I was counting the days to August when I'd be going to Butlins, Skegness, with my friend Mandy. I felt desperately in need of a break from work. My job wasn't stretching me at all, but I hid my burning desire for something more in a brilliant ongoing act of conformity. One night I dreamt I was getting on with my boring work while all the time I was crying. Sobbing out loud, simply howling, the tears rushing unchecked down my face. But the people around me were just carrying on working as if they couldn't see or hear my tears. I continued to work efficiently. I filed invoices, stamped envelopes, typed lists and letters; carried on doing the things I did on an ordinary day at work. But all the time I was crying like the Queen of Sorrows. And no one knew. I awoke, feeling disturbed.

Prompted by my 'crying' dream, I went to the library and read the careers reference books. What was I interested in? People. Writing. So how about writing features on social issues? Journalism? Yes, but that job needed an 'outgoing personality' and shyness would hold me back. Oh, damn, damn, damn my shyness! Need O and A levels? Need to go to college? Yes, well maybe I could do that? Hang on, better see if I can write first.

I dipped into my savings and enrolled for a correspondence course in 'Modern Journalism'. While waiting for my first lesson to arrive, I wrote an article on what it was like to be a teenager in the sixties, about the lack of understanding and guidance, the pressures, double standards, hypocrisy that faced us, including some criticisms of Christianity as it is often practised. I sent my article to the local paper and was amazed when a staff photographer arrived at our house. I posed shyly for him. So there I was a few days later, smiling out from a page in the paper beneath the headlines '"LET'S BRIDGE THAT AGE GAP", SAYS TEENAGER'. Letters both praising and criticising what I'd written appeared in further editions, and also arrived on the doormat. I'd never expected such 'fame' and was flattered, embarrassed and amused by it.

The disco was crowded and noisy as usual. Feeling bleary-eyed with gin, I almost didn't recognise my friend from Rainbow Land days. That girl at the next table, heavily made-up, sad-looking, chain-smoking: my God, it was Carrie, my childhood friend who'd dreamt of going to art school.

'Jean! Well, stop looking so bloody surprised. You've changed a lot, too, you know.'

On impulse I invited Carrie on a weekend in Blackpool that I was planning with Mandy. She said she'd love to come.

It was great being with Carrie again on that holiday. Mandy brought along her old friend Jane who was a fairly reserved type (I think by nature rather than by shyness). Later, Mandy told me how Jane was disgusted with the way Carrie and I laughed and carried on 'like a pair of silly school kids'. But it had all been innocent, rollicking good fun. It's just as well Carrie and I did manage to snatch back, at least briefly, something of our childhood because I don't think either of us found much to laugh about in the years that were swiftly to follow.

Oh, Carrie, did you ever have time, amidst your teenage marriage, pregnancies and painful divorce, to remember a day long ago in Rainbow Land when the sun shone through leaves making criss-cross patterns on our arms and legs while we lay in the grass sharing secrets? What happened to your Art School dream?

I kept asking myself what had gone wrong with a society where violence was escalating? What had gone wrong with a society

227

where the odds were rapidly increasing against adolescents living through their teen years without getting pregnant, suicidal, running away, or becoming addicted to drink, drugs or a cult? What had gone wrong with a society where too many parts of Teensville, that 'wonderful world of the young', were becoming littered with wrecked young lives?

But I must have believed there was something wrong with me rather than society when I went on that Butlins holiday with Mandy a few weeks later. Or I wouldn't have thought my unhappiness should be anything to do with doctors, would I?

She has never, since leaving school, been in a job or situation which has totally occupied her intellectual capabilities thus leading to a situation of self-centred analysis and concern.

I do not think there is any evidence of this girl being schizophrenic — I believe this is a girl of above-average intelligence, dissatisfied with her life style and thus devoting a lot of time trying to figure out a religious or philosophical ideology to cover her life style.

Dr Copeland

PART THREE

A SELF TO RECOVER

They thought death was worth it, but I
Have a self to recover, a queen.

Sylvia Plath

CHAPTER EIGHTEEN

TIME PASSED. TIME ALWAYS passed, despite everything, and it had passed quicker than I'd realised. Dr Shaw at the day hospital made me aware of that when he called me into the office upstairs, motioned for me to sit on the chair opposite his desk near the window, and asked, 'What date is it?'

I knew the day was Thursday – I would be going to Vera's for tea as I did every Thursday – and I knew it was May or June in 1972 but I couldn't elaborate further. I gazed out of the window across the grounds where a group of elderly female patients, led by two nurses, shuffled along in single file, each wearing a shapeless cotton dress and old-fashioned straw sunbonnet with a large brim. I wondered if they were on Largactil. That would explain the bonnets, as patients on that drug are often hypersensitive to sunlight. My medication had been switched back to Melleril after my continued complaints about the effects of Largactil. Not that it helped. I felt as dreadful and drowsy on either.

'I'm waiting for you to tell me the *full* date,' Dr Shaw said, rapping with his pen on the desk to regain my attention. 'Now, come along, Jean. What have you got to say to me?'

I had nothing at all to say to him. It seemed pointless trying to explain how you lose track of time because it doesn't matter a toss what day or month or year it is when your mind is in a drugged torpor and each dark day that looms ahead merges into an endless tunnel.

'How long have you been depressed?'

'Dr Copeland doesn't think I'm clinically depressed.'

His face tightened into a frown and I realised telling him

this was probably as unwise as my telling Sister Oldroyd when Dr Prior had said I didn't have to go to OT.

'*I* think you're depressed,' he said firmly, placing much emphasis on the 'I'. 'How long ago was it when you were in Thornville?'

'I don't know,' I replied sleepily. My after-dinner drugs were taking their toll and I was too tired to answer questions.

'That's not good enough, Jean. Try to remember.'

'It must've been at least a year ago,' I offered vaguely. 'Or maybe longer. Could've been about two years, I think.'

'At least a year ago? Or could have been two years? Think again, Jean. Come on. How long ago?'

'I ... I don't know,' I said, trying to stifle a yawn.

'I'll tell you how long ago it was,' Dr Shaw said, rustling the papers on his desk. 'It was three and half years ago.'

'Was it?' I stared at him in shocked surprise. How could three and half years of my life disappear just like that? What had gone wrong with time? What had gone wrong with everything? What had gone wrong with *me*? I gazed out of the window again, trying to digest this information. My God, it was three and half years ago! I'd been a teenager then. I'd never be a teenager again. I'd never have those three and half years back.

Dr Shaw rapped with his pen for my attention again.

'You've been attending this day hospital for about eighteen months. It was three and half years ago when you were an in-patient. Over three years,' he said, tapping three times with his pen, 'in which time you've been seen by Dr Sugden, Dr Prior, Dr Dean, Dr Armstrong, Dr Copeland and myself. Haven't you?' Starting from Dr Sugden on his thumb, he had waggled each finger in turn as he named each of these psychiatrists.

'Dr Dean?' I said, looking at the finger which had waggled for Dr Dean and wondering if this name had been thrown in to test me. 'No, I've never seen a Dr Dean.'

He looked through the papers in front of him, then back at me.

'Anyway, the point I am making is that during the past three and half years, you've seen several doctors, been given ECT, drugs, and participated in occupational therapy. Haven't you?'

'Yes,' I agreed.

'And we're still not moving much, are we? Perhaps we should try a course of ECT.'

I shuddered. I still perceived ECT as a damaging experience that had left me definitely emotionally, and probably physically, scarred. My distressing memories of the treatment were something I would have to learn to live with. Always.

'I'm not having any more ECT,' I said.

'We've been trying to help you for a long time, haven't we?'

'Yes,' I said.

'Why, then, during all that time, have your parents never once made enquiries about you and your treatment?'

I shrugged my shoulders.

'Take your mother, for instance. What's she playing at?' he asked, thumping his desk. 'She should have been on the phone and up here long ago, demanding to know what's going on. Doesn't she care?'

Here it was again. The all-too-familiar mother-blaming attitude – although, Lord knows, maybe I was guilty, too, of blaming her for more than she deserved. But was Dr Shaw saying what he *really* felt, or just wanting to see how I'd react if he pretended to be angry with my mother? I tried to push this thought from my mind because I knew only too well how difficult, how frustrating, how damn near impossible it was to achieve meaningful communication with staff while trying to decide whether or not they were talking in a certain way only to observe your reaction to it. Perhaps I ought to take them at face value more? Maybe Mr Jordan really did agree with wife-beating and meant it when he said he'd hit my mother if in my dad's situation? Maybe Dr Shaw really was angry with my mother now?

My eyes had wandered to the window again while I'd been trying to sort out my thoughts about all this. A sparrow flew past and hopped from branch to branch of a tree, then soared up into the sky to become a dot on the horizon before disappearing far away. I wished I was far away too. Far away from the hospital. Far away from the whole stupid mess. Oh, I wished ...

'Jean, look at me,' Dr Shaw said in his schoolteacher's voice. 'Stop drifting away into daydreams and listen to me.'

'I'm sorry,' I said. 'I'm listening.'

And I did listen. Listened as he bombarded me with questions which bore no relation whatsoever to the reasons I'd sought psychiatric 'help'. 'Do you hear voices?' 'Tell me, Jean, do you ever think things that are obscene?' 'Do you ever see things that other people don't seem able to see?' 'Do you sometimes feel other people might be able to hear or control your thoughts?'

I listened until my head spun with his irrelevant questions that in no way connected with my experiences. I wondered if he'd got my case notes mixed up with someone else's. Didn't he believe me when I said no, I wasn't having, had never had, auditory or visual hallucinations? Should I be having them? And, no, to all the other questions. God, I was tired. I stared out of the window again, wondering if sometimes patients confessed to anything if they thought it might end the interrogation.

'I don't think we're getting anywhere, are we?'

'No, we're not,' I agreed.

'Why hasn't your mother asked to see us?' he said again.

'I don't know. Maybe because she doesn't like psychiatrists.'

'A lot of people don't like psychiatrists. And you know why that is, don't you?' he said, pausing for effect and leaning forwards as if about to impart some deep words of wisdom to me. 'That's because psychiatrists get at the truth.'

I sighed, and stifled another yawn.

'Would your mother see me if I sent her an appointment?'

'Yes, I think so,' I said.

'You may go now,' he said, looking at his watch.

As I left the office, I thought about Dr Shaw's claim that

psychiatrists 'get at the truth'. Reaction-testing? No, I didn't think so this time. I decided this was what he honestly believed.

About two weeks later, my mother, wearing her short skirt and blonde wig, sat next to me opposite Dr Shaw while Mr Jordan was seated to our right.

'Do you mind if I smoke?' she asked.

'No, not at all,' said Dr Shaw.

'That's me only bad habit and, even so, I get nowt but criticism for it at home,' she said, lighting a cigarette and holding it between nicotine-stained fingers. She looked away from Dr Shaw each time he spoke to her and was obviously self-conscious. My sympathy for her embarrassment was tainted with anger at the way she tried to present herself as the family martyr, the one who was constantly criticised but never the cause of family squabbles. My anger manifested itself in fidgets, puffs and tuts until Dr Shaw asked me to leave the room.

Later that day, Mr Jordan laughed about my 'hostile' behaviour towards my mother during the interview.

'Oh heck, was it so obvious?'

'It was understandable,' he said, 'so don't worry about it.'

He leant back in his chair, looking thoughtful. 'I'll tell you what's *really* puzzling about you. It's that you're so different from what one could expect, considering what I know about your background.'

'What do you mean?' I asked. I didn't think he knew very much about my background.

'Do you know what schizophrenia is?' he asked.

I wondered why he'd suddenly changed the subject. I trotted out the usual lay person's definition: 'Isn't it summat to do with a split personality?'

'A maladjusted personality.'

'My friend's sister's been diagnosed as schizophrenic. It's awful. Her whole life's destroyed.'

Thinking about Donna made me feel sad. Schizophrenia

seemed the most devastating illness and I was glad I hadn't got that.

'Anyway, what did you mean about me being different from what you'd expect knowing about my background?' I asked.

'Oh, a few things,' he said, 'but never mind.'

'You've got me curious now.'

'Well, didn't you once tell me your brother needed an extra year in primary school because he was a slow learner? Quite different from you, isn't he? And it wouldn't be surprising, with your home situation, if you were acting irresponsibly, stealing, behaving promiscuously, ending up pregnant. And yet you're not at all likely to do things like that. You've got principles, which I admire.'

'Hey, steady on. I'm no angel,' I said, smiling.

How very different, how quite the opposite, were Mr Jordan's and Dr Copeland's approach from that of the other psychiatric staff I'd encountered. Whether they were right or wrong, they certainly helped to shore up my confidence and self-worth at a time in my life when there was much to destroy it. I was sorry to hear that Mr Jordan was about to be transferred to one of the wards.

Sister Speight, a stern-faced, bossy woman, replaced Mr Jordan at the day hospital.

'Right, Vera,' Sister Speight said. 'Off you go upstairs to see Dr Shaw, but first take these beakers back into the kitchen.'

Vera must have heard the first instruction but not the second. She was halfway up the stairs when Sister Speight shouted at her.

'Vera! Vera Dixon! Come down this minute! Are you deaf? Now, what did I tell you to do before going upstairs?'

With heavy heart at seeing Vera, a wife and mother in her forties, being treated like a naughty child, I joined the patients in the therapy room, where a sleepy atmosphere prevailed.

Sister Speight came in, waving some sheets of paper, and clapped her hands for attention. 'Let's have some signs of life in here. It's like a morgue. We're going to have a sing-song.'

Soon after Vera returned to the therapy room, Sister Speight's sing-song was interrupted because Dr Shaw wanted to take our photographs. He was keen on doing this. We went outside and dutifully lined up and posed for him by the flowerbeds.

'Aidan, put your arm around Jean,' Dr Shaw directed. I supposed it was because Dr Shaw liked these photos to portray a 'one big happy family' image.

Aidan looked embarrassed. He was a shy, quiet young man who seemed to live in a world of his own.

'Come on, Aidan, put your arm round her,' Dr Shaw persisted.

Aidan glanced at me and blushed. Everyone was waiting. Stiffly, Aidan's arm extended to hang awkwardly around my shoulder.

'Good, that will do,' Dr Shaw said, focusing his camera. 'Now, smile everybody. You as well, Marlene and Georgina. Say cheese.'

On our way back inside, Marlene said to me, 'He's a fucking weird creep.'

'Who?'

'Dr Shaw, of course. Making you and Aidan pose like a courting couple for his photo. It's sick if you ask me. The other day he got me to sit on the floor with Don Parker and he told Don to put his arm round me. What does he do with all these photos anyway? I'd like to get hold of his camera and shove it up his arse.'

We returned to the therapy room where, led by an arm-waving Sister Speight, we sang 'Onward Christian Soldiers'. Dad once said that, when he was in prison, the Salvation Army came and sang 'Bless This House'. It amused me to think of singing to prisoners: 'Bless these walls so firm and stout, keeping want and trouble out'. What we were doing now seemed no less ironic, but Sister Speight looked deadly serious. Vera, Georgina and I kept exchanging glances and giggling behind our song sheets like naughty schoolchildren. One aid to survival in the mental hospital world was to wring as much humour as possible out of each absurd situation.

A small group of us once frightened a museum attendant on an outing. We were bored and looking for an exit so we could slip out and go for a coffee, but we wandered off down the wrong corridor.

'You can't get out that way,' the attendant informed us. 'You'll have to go back along the corridor, turn right and go up the stairs then along the corridor to go down the far stairs which bring you out near the main entrance.'

'Oh, tickle to that,' said Marlene. 'Surely there's a quicker way out.' She mopped her forehead and waved her arms dramatically. 'Let us out. We need to get out quick or we'll be having a funny do. We're from High Royds.'

The attendant immediately produced some keys and all but shoved us out of a small back exit a few yards from where we'd been standing. No one was going to be allowed to have a funny do in his museum. Outside in the street, we doubled up laughing. 'Did you see the look on his face?' Marlene asked with a chuckle. 'He couldn't let us out quick enough when I mentioned High Royds.'

Even the hospital parrot had a sense of humour. In part of the grounds surrounding the hospital there was a small aviary which housed, among other birds, Popsy the parrot whose party piece was to say 'O be joyful' to the watching groups of depressed patients.

'O be joyful,' Popsy said as Georgina stuck her face near the mesh to get a closer look.

'Don't you "O be joyful" me,' Georgina said crossly.

'O be joyful. O be joyful. O be joyful,' the parrot squawked, running backwards and forwards along its perch.

'You horrible creature. I'll wring your neck if you don't shut up,' Georgina said, sounding as if she meant it, but then she turned to me with a smile. 'Oh, listen to me arguing with a bloody parrot. I'm so miserable and bad-tempered today, I don't know what to do.'

'What to do? What to do? O be joyful,' the parrot suggested.

We both laughed.

Mike was sending me long letters with news cuttings and pictures about life in New Zealand. He'd got a well-paid job with a car manufacturer, had never been so well off financially, was living it up at champagne parties and said it was really great out there. But reading between the lines I knew he was homesick. In some of his letters he begged me to join him, offering to pay my fare. He kept telling me he loved me and wanted to marry me.

And he didn't even know me.

CHAPTER NINETEEN

I IGNORED THEM FOR a long time but, yes, they were there, these questions in the recesses of my mind, like tiny seeds hidden beneath the soil. Lately they had started growing, spreading their tendrils and thrusting their way up through the darkness to the surface. Despite my drowsiness, I was becoming increasingly critical of psychiatry. How could 'helping' include abusing people's minds and bodies, inflicting pain and humiliation, indoctrinating people into believing themselves inadequate, while fostering a dependency on mental hospitals and drugs?

'I'm sick of this hospital,' I blurted out the minute I was seated at Dr Copeland's desk on what proved to be the last occasion I would see him. 'Is it part of the staff's training to view us as something less than human beings?'

'I'm not doing that, am I? Why are you angry with me?'

'It's not you,' I admitted. He was the one psychiatrist I knew who least deserved this kind of criticism. I twisted my fingers nervously. 'It's not just one incident or one person,' I tried to explain. 'It's your ... your profession. Psychiatry!' I spat out the word vehemently. 'There's something ... something wrong with it,' I said, fumbling to find the right words from my half-formed thoughts.

Dr Copeland smiled. 'Yes, and some of us would like to change things. But who or what has annoyed you?'

'I've told you it's nobody in particular. It's lots of things.'

I searched my mind for examples, but could only launch into recounting bitterly my initiation into the mental hospital world on Thornville.

'OK, so you had a bad experience on one of the wards, but don't judge the whole hospital by that.'

'I'm not,' I said. 'It's also what I've experienced over the years since, and what I've seen happening to other people. It's now as well, all the time, and it's not just ... it's got something to do with ... with the whole system.'

I didn't know whether to laugh or cry. I felt I was teetering on the brink of an important revelation but, having finally grasped a bit of truth, I couldn't digest or express it.

'You're feeling angry today, Jean,' Dr Copeland observed, lighting a cigarette.

'Yes, too right I am. Patient's symptoms took the form of anger today.' I gave a sarcastic laugh. 'So why don't you increase my tablets or send me for ECT?' I wouldn't have dared say that to Dr Shaw. I could only say it to Dr Copeland because I could trust him not to do that.

I gazed at the sky through the window, feeling as though I was watching the clouds through prison bars.

'I feel like smashing every window in this bloody hospital,' I said, suppressed anger crackling inside me and shooting off sparks.

'Go ahead if it'll make you feel any better,' Dr Copeland muttered sleepily, 'but then you'll have to pay for them.' He yawned and stretched.

'You know something?' I went on heedlessly, my bottled-up emotions bobbing close to the surface. 'If you're not mad when you first come into this hospital, you've little chance of not being after a while.'

'That applies to the staff, too,' Dr Copeland replied.

We both sat silently for a while, then I said: 'I really don't understand how I got myself into all this.'

Dr Copeland leant forward in his chair, resting his chin on his hand propped up by his elbow.

'Jean, didn't you once tell me that it was *you* who first asked to see a psychiatrist?'

I nodded.

'What exactly did you say to him?'

'I told him I thought I was going insane.'

He sighed. 'Asking to see a psychiatrist and telling him you think you're going insane.' He closed his eyes and ran his fingers across his forehead. 'Jesus, what a clever thing to do! Like voluntarily putting your head on the chopping block, don't you think?'

'With hindsight, yes,' I replied. 'But I felt I needed help and asking to see a psychiatrist seemed a sensible thing to do.'

'What kind of help did you expect?'

'Not the so-called help I got,' I said, bitterly.

'But what did you expect?'

'I don't know. Maybe I wanted him to reassure me that I *wasn't* going insane. I needed someone to talk to and I was scared he wouldn't take me seriously.'

'So you told him you thought you were going insane to make sure he'd sit up and listen to you? Sounds like you were playing a very dangerous game.'

I hung my head and thought about it carefully before answering.

'No, that's not fair. It wasn't a game,' I said finally. 'I'd been full of conflicts and confusion, and so dissatisfied with life, for a long time. I didn't know where to turn. Asking to see a psychiatrist was my cry for help. And did you know it takes courage to do that? But how, please tell me how, am I supposed to understand what happened next? Once inside, nothing made sense any more: strong drugs right away, too drowsy to think straight, then ECT only a few days later ...' The words were rushing out now, hot and angry. 'It all happened so quickly and I was sucked in too deep to get out. It was like ... like being crushed with a steamroller. God, how I wish I'd never made that decision to see a psychiatrist, but I was a mixed-up teenager and I thought ... I honestly thought I was being ... sensible.'

I nearly choked on the word 'sensible' as painful memories flooded my mind, drenching me in self-pity for having paid such a high price for being 'sensible'. I was holding back so many tears and feelings now that they were rumbling in my stomach and causing painful contractions in my chest and throat.

'I wonder what patients expect of us,' Dr Copeland said, stroking his chin. I thought I detected pity in his eyes when he said again, though very gently this time: 'What did you expect?'

'I don't know,' I said with a deep sigh as I managed to compose myself. 'I just don't know.'

The consultation was over. I was leaving Dr Copeland's office when he called me back.

'Can I give you some off-the-record advice?' he asked. He was looking down at his desk as if talking to that.

'OK. I'm listening.'

'Get away from this hospital. I know it's not easy, but can't you try to get a job and your own flat?' His tone was quiet, gentle, almost pleading. 'You *can* see, Jean, can't you, why it's so important that you get right away from all this?' He paused, looked up at me and spoke louder, firmer, urgently. 'For Christ's sake, Jean, get away from here. Before it's too late!'

Dr Copeland left the hospital and I heard from staff that he had given up psychiatry to become a GP. Dr Shaw informed me that I'd be seeing him more in future, an announcement which filled me with dismay. Sister Speight was replaced by a charge nurse called Tony, a pleasant young man in his late twenties. Georgina took a massive overdose and went into a coma. And so life (or whatever it should be called) at the hospital, went on.

After Dr Copeland left, I did make some attempt to 'get away' before it was 'too late', but felt trapped. I applied for jobs as a dental receptionist, a typist, and at a hairdresser's washing hair and sweeping up, but job-hunting seemed pointless. On application forms, or at interviews, how could I explain my long gap of unemployment, and my present situation? How could I get references? Who would want to employ a drugged mental patient?

I scanned the newspaper for accommodation but this, too, seemed beyond my reach. How could I support myself financially? Nikki, an acquaintance of Jackie, phoned me one evening. I'd never met Nikki but she explained she needed someone to share her flat and Jackie had told her I was looking for a place.

'Well, I *was*, but I've stopped looking for now because … because I'm unemployed at the moment,' I explained.

'Oh, I didn't realise you were between jobs, but never mind. We could meet for a coffee if you like and perhaps decide about sharing the flat for later. What kind of work do you do?'

'Office work,' I replied, 'but I haven't worked for some time.' I hesitated, then plunged in. 'I'm a patient at a psychiatric day hospital.'

'Oh!'

'Didn't Jackie tell you?'

There was a long, awkward silence.

'Oh, I … er, I see. No, I didn't know.'

Another long pause. There was no sign now of her initial friendliness. Her obvious unease was greater than I'd anticipated. I might as well have told her I'd got bubonic plague.

Before going to bed I looked at myself in the wardrobe mirror. I was not the fat girl I had been on my discharge from Thornville, for I had long since regained my slim, pre-hospital figure. But it was still a dull, heavy-lidded, pale, lifeless creature who stared back at me. Where had I gone? Somewhere in the cellars of my mind there was a dusty memory of how it had felt to be awake and alive. I remembered a girl on a swing in a park – it made me want to cry.

I sat on the bed and tipped my dosage of pills from their little plastic containers into my hand. Valium pills were yellow, amitriptyline were red, and the white ones were Melleril, and Kemedrin. Resisting a sudden urge to throw them on the floor, I forced them down my throat with a large gulp of water and winced. For a while now my pills had seemed to be sticking, causing a tight band of pain in my chest that hurt more each time I swallowed.

I lay on the bed staring at the ceiling while Brian's loud music from the record player downstairs battered my brain. My head felt heavy, groggy, and my stomach acknowledged the arrival of the latest pills with a queasy flutter. It was as if, after years of daily drug-taking, my mind and body were now pleading in unison, 'No more. Oh, please no more.'

Existing on pills, going to the hospital, living with my family, being painfully shy, feeling constantly tired, lacking energy and motivation; all these things were getting me down. And now there was this disturbing, restless feeling reminding me that it was of the utmost importance to do something before it was too late. The problem was I'd no idea what this 'something' should be. Leave home, get a flat, get a job, get away from the hospital … Yes, yes, yes, Dr Copeland. But how? I felt I'd lost the skills for 'normal' living (if I'd ever had them).

I pulled the raggy, dirty bedcovers over my head, feeling too exhausted to have a wash or clean my teeth. I lay awkwardly in the lumpy, unmade bed, trying as always to avoid the spring that was protruding through the mattress, but it caught the seat of my pyjamas and ripped them when I tugged free. With my fingers stuck in my ears to block out the pounding music, I sought refuge in sleep. I wasn't feeling very well tonight. So what was new?

CHAPTER TWENTY

SAVED BY THE BELL. My alarm clock rescued me from a nightmare in which once again I was being held down firmly by white-coated men who were about to shoot electric currents into my brain. I leant over to stop it and lay back down. I still wasn't feeling well and may have been tempted to stay in bed if it hadn't been my brother's day off. I lay staring at the ceiling, with my arm stretched across my forehead, until I'd no time for breakfast. Then I got up, had a quick wash, pulled on my jeans and a T-shirt, swallowed a handful of pills and set off for the day hospital.

I felt sick during the bus journey so had to get off a few stops early. I walked the rest of the way and was still feeling a bit fragile when Tony greeted me with the news that my presence was required immediately at a Case Review Meeting. I'd never attended one but I knew from staff and patients something of what to expect. The room would be full of students and others, all sitting around me making notes, staring, observing my reactions to questions. Tony saw me pull a face and said kindly, 'You'll be OK, it's nothing to worry about,' as he led me to the office upstairs.

'Tell us about the church you used to go to,' Dr Shaw said while my audience stared.

How long ago it seemed since I'd gone to church with Jackie and sung hymns with a joyful heart before the shadows descended. How could they understand? Why should I try to explain?

Andy, the young friendly student nurse who was presently

based at the day hospital, piped up, 'You're all right about religion now. I know you can see it from both sides because I've heard you talk about it.'

I turned to Andy who was sitting behind me.

'But it's seeing it from both sides like that which caused the conflicts,' I pointed out. 'If I hadn't seen it from both sides, I'd have been able to either carry on being a Christian or become an atheist, depending on which side I could see it from.'

'Turn round and talk to me,' Dr Shaw said firmly.

Dr Shaw's questions made me uncomfortable. As always, they were selective; for example, I wasn't asked about my father's adulterous affairs – not that I wanted to be.

'Tell me about your mother's affair.'

'Has your mother had affairs in the past?'

'Has your mother slept with a lot of men?'

I supposed if I snapped at them to mind their own business, my anger would be seen as a symptom of illness. They can ask me anything, I thought, to write about in that manila file with my name on it, then use the partial truths and fictions it contains, all the distortions of their blinkered medical perspective, as proof of who knows what. *Stop it, Jean, that's a sick way to think.* They only wanted to help, so I should try to cooperate with them. But, Lord, I'd been co-operating for years and look where it had got me …

I tried to answer questions about my mother honestly, although I felt guilty and disloyal for doing so to these note-taking strangers. And I tried to talk about myself with an openness that rendered me vulnerable. I did this, even though seeing a psychiatrist in the first place to talk about myself now seemed the biggest mistake of my life.

My throat was parched. I couldn't swallow. Twice earlier I'd asked Dr Shaw if I could have a glass of water and each time he'd just smiled inanely and carried on with his questions as if my request wasn't worth acknowledging. Now my mouth was so dry I could hardly speak, my tongue got in the way of my words and I sounded as if I had a speech impediment. An excessively dry mouth was one of the side effects of my drugs, and I expect nervousness at having to speak in front of all these people was accentuating it. Tony stood up and left the room as I struggled on. After a short while, he returned with a glass of water for me. I was very grateful.

'Do you hear voices?' Dr Shaw asked.

'Not like what you mean. Not audible voices.'

'Not audible voices? Well, what kind of voices do you hear?'

'I don't hear voices, but I mean sometimes your own thoughts are like voices, aren't they? A kind of dialogue in your mind.'

'Are they really?' he said, looking interested.

I wished I hadn't said that. Had it made me sound schizophrenic? I'd been taught at Sunday school to listen to the 'still small voice' of conscience, the God-part inside us. After the loss of my religious beliefs I'd perceived this 'voice' as a part of my thoughts, but I didn't mean a 'voice' literally.

'Everybody thinks that way at times, don't they?' I said nervously.

'What way?'

'That your thoughts are like voices inside you.'

A stony silence. Damn it, I was making it worse.

'But I can't *hear* them. I only mean "voices" in a metaphorical sense,' I said in a hoarse voice that ended in a whisper.

It's no good trying to explain, I thought. He probably even thinks the pop song by the Paper Dolls titled 'Something Here In My Heart (Keeps A-Tellin' Me No)' is about mental illness. I picked up my glass with a shaky hand and took a gulp of water. The note-takers were scribbling away and Dr Shaw was wearing his funny little smile. Train people to look for symptoms of illness and they'll find something sick about the desk and chairs if they expect to, I thought angrily. What a bunch of lemons!

'Do you ever wonder if people can hear your thoughts?'

'No, and sometimes it's a jolly good job they can't,' I replied with feeling.

A few chuckles rippled around the room diffusing the heavy atmosphere, but only for a moment.

It was *awful*. I felt as if I was being interrogated, found guilty of mental illness and the sentence was the destruction of my credibility and self-esteem. I can't take this much longer, they're pushing me over the edge, I thought, while another voice inside me (not an audible voice, you understand) was saying: No, you're wrong to think this way, Jean, they only want to help and now you're getting paranoid.

No, it wasn't me. This was enough to drive the sanest person crazy.

OK, I think they really might be only wanting to help, I decided finally, but the problem was that they were *so dangerously wrong*. And I was one of the casualties of this narrow-minded, medically orientated perspective, one who had been placed in grave danger because of their wrongness.

'Why did you first see a psychiatrist?' Dr Shaw asked.

I needed more time to think that one out for myself. Was being caught up in conflicts and confusion about religion and life a medical problem? But life had seemed meaningless and empty; depression was a medical problem, wasn't it?

'Come along, Jean. Would you like to try to tell us why?'

'Because I thought ... I thought I was depressed.'

'You *thought* you were depressed? And weren't you?'

'Well, yes, I suppose so in a way, but ... but, no, not *really*,' I said.

'You were depressed but you weren't? That doesn't make sense, does it?'

'Yes it does,' I said defensively. 'I mean ... I mean I wasn't *fully* depressed.'

'Oh? And have you ever been *fully* depressed?'

'Yes. In Thornville Ward. I never knew depression before then. Not what I'd call depression now. I didn't even realise until then that it was possible to feel so ...' My voice wavered.

'Did going into hospital help you?'

Hadn't he heard what I'd just said? 'How could it have helped? How could it have done anything other than make me worse? And that's all psychiatry has ever done for me,' I blurted out, as I glanced up accusingly at the others, then back at Dr Shaw. 'You start treating people in ways that can be harmful, without knowing enough ... without even knowing *anything* about the person you're treating. Without understanding a single thing ...'

My voice trembled as I came close to tears. But I wouldn't cry in front of them. I wouldn't. The hurt turned to anger. Dr Shaw had a sort of I-know-how-you-feel-dear smile on his face and I was sure they'd heard all this before from many other poor, sick nerve cases. I suspected they believed these kind of criticisms came only from patients who lacked 'insight'. Didn't it occur to them that hurt and angry, even confused or sick, patients could be right about some things? If only they would tear up their goddamn notepads, unshackle their minds from their training, forget about the textbooks they'd read and just *listen* and *hear*. Oh, wasn't there at least one person among them who could understand what was happening at this hospital and see that it was wrong?

I glanced at the sea of faces around me; all eyes were staring intently at me. There were about twelve people in the room, mostly males, seated around the desk where Dr Shaw sat facing me. I turned and looked at Andy sitting behind me. His fresh open face looked serious, thoughtful. I shifted my gaze to the person on his right and held it there for a moment. And then on to the next person, and the next. And the next. All the way round the room, looking steadily at each person in turn for a while. Nobody spoke. Most of them looked uncomfortable under my gaze and lowered their eyes, shuffled their feet or coughed nervously. I got a kind of fleeting, perverse pleasure out of this despite my growing anxiety that I was finally cracking up.

I rested my eyes longest on a young bearded man who I thought looked caring, as if trying to understand. And he didn't look away. But I realised that I was probably seeing him as I wanted to see him. Finally, I looked back at Dr Shaw, then down at the floor. Afraid and alone.

I was locked in a nightmare from which I couldn't awaken, trapped in a horror film and cast in the star part as victim. A role which would have to be played out right to the tragic finale. Or would it? Perhaps I could still say 'NO!' and not allow it to happen. I must shatter the screen, make good my escape and rewrite the script.

'Right, thank you, Jean,' Dr Shaw said, bringing the session to an end.

I remained seated a moment longer, thinking things out.

Dr Shaw coughed. 'It's time for you to go now.'

Yes, it's time for me to go now, I thought. And please, dear God, don't let it be too late.

The room seemed thick with tension and deathly quiet as I stood up. Then Andy sprang to his feet, patted my shoulder and, smiling warmly, said, 'See ya later, kiddo. Tarra.' I liked him for that.

'Has anybody got any questions?' I heard Dr Shaw ask just after I closed the door on leaving.

Yes, *me*. I've got some questions, I thought. I've got so many questions that I've been ignoring for far too long.

The first thing I must do had suddenly become so obvious to me and I knew that this time I must see it through to the end. Were being drowsy, depressed, lacking in energy and motivation, symptoms of illness or side effects of drugs? It seemed that outlets for my feelings, whether through writing, talking, tears or whatever, had all been, to a large extent, blocked off by the drugs I'd taken for years. It couldn't be healthy, this pressing down of emotions. It was as if I'd packed them tightly into a bottle and pushed a cork in. What would happen if the cork shot out? Would feelings that had been contained for so long erupt like a volcano if released? Perhaps I really was sick and perhaps I did need the drugs, but I had to find out. Frozen in stone, buried before my time, what had I got to lose anyway? I decided to take the cork out myself.

The next morning, a Saturday, I went round the house opening drawers and cupboards, gathering together all the pills accumulated over the years through missing just one dose every so often, then I added these to my present supply, and emptied the whole lot down the toilet. But several flushes later, they were obstinately remaining at the bottom of the toilet bowl; miserable reminders of those years of my life that I wanted to flush away along with the pills.

I scooped out a soggy, yellow handful of Valium pills, but still couldn't flush the other pills away. Damn it! I fished out the rest and loaded them back into their plastic containers. There had recently been an advertising campaign urging people to get rid of old pills safely by taking them to a chemist. With this in mind, I set off out.

On my way back from the chemist, I had a strong urge to cut my hair. It was straight and very long, hanging loosely to my waist, and I'd worn it like that since I was about sixteen. Sure that I'd make a mess with the scissors myself, I called in at the local hairdresser's who said they could fit me in right away for a trim.

'I want a lot cutting off,' I explained. 'I'd like it to just below my ears.'

'Oh, but you've got such lovely long hair. Are you sure you want so much cutting off?'

'Yes. Quite sure.'

Snip, snip, snip … A part of me, formed over the years, fell away in seconds. The three other hairdressers and the girl who did the shampooing stopped what they were doing to silently stand and watch, though they couldn't have understood the solemnity of the occasion. Cutting off my hair had somehow got connected in my mind with cutting off my past; a kind of symbolic ritual. I don't know what gave me that idea. A character in Rosamond Lehmann's *Dusty Answer* has her long hair cut short for much the same reason, but I didn't read that novel until several years later.

Back outside, I breathed in the fresh air, blowing away the cobwebs in my brain. How strange it felt to toss my head and not feel the weight of long, thick hair. Change was in the air. I could feel it, breathe it, smell it and taste it on my lips. High in the sky the sun was peeping out from behind a grey cloud and, for the first time in how long, I felt exhilarated. No more drugs. After years of being a zombie, I was coming back to life again. It's like being reborn, I thought excitedly.

Lying in bed that night with no bottles of pills beside my bed for the first time in years, but feeling restless, unable to sleep, some of my earlier optimism about being reborn faded as I began to glimpse something of the struggle that lay ahead.

It was going to be a painful birth.

CHAPTER TWENTY-ONE

I DIDN'T KNOW I was a drug addict. I thought drug addicts were illicit-drug users who belonged to the shady world of dealers and pushers, shifty transactions in discos and bars, fixes in lavatories; and I was never part of that scene.

I awoke early on Sunday morning, feeling shaky after a few hours of restless sleep. As the day wore on I felt irritable and Brian's behaviour grated on my nerves more than usual. Tomorrow I would have to face the day hospital. I went to bed early.

My mind raced here and there, raking up incidents from the past few years. When I eventually fell asleep, it was as if my brain was processing stored-up information like a computer. Every so often I awoke with a start, sat up and thought: Yes, that's right! Most of these insights had been kicking around for a long time, at least on a cerebral level, but somehow never before hitting me on this deeper level with such shattering intensity. My thoughts and criticisms of psychiatry, formed gradually and tentatively over the years, now hung forcefully together as a dazzling confirmation of truth which must be acted on without further delay.

Throughout the night I kept waking to flashes of insight into myself, my family situation and psychiatry, especially psychiatry. Clear, painful, disturbing, illuminating glimpses of truth. Although I sensed I was wobbling precariously near to an emotional upheaval which might cause me to lose my balance, I had never experienced a state that was more self-revealing. By morning I felt weak and exhausted, but amidst the hovering fears and ambiguities that threatened to clog up my mind, two things stood out with soul-shaking clarity: I had to get away from the hospital and I had to leave home.

I wanted to do both things immediately, but first I had to find suitable accommodation and I needed hospital staff to back up my attempt to get a job. But no longer would I delay plans to achieve these two objectives now that I'd taken the first step to freedom by discarding the drugs.

When I arrived at the day hospital, Geoff stared at me with unconcealed disappointment. 'Oh! You've cut off your long, beautiful hair,' he said, looking as if he was going to cry.

The day passed uneventfully. I felt reasonably together, although a bit preoccupied and I almost forgot to pour Arnold's coffee. On the bus home I began sweating and shaking but managed to control the ripples of panic which threatened to take hold.

When I arrived home Brian began talking about people 'taking over the country'. My father, too, believed this and, to my dismay, had become a member of the National Front.

Oh God, not today, I thought. I can't face this kind of talking today. I pictured Samuel sitting in the hospital library, his face contorted in painful recollection as he cried out, 'I hate the Nazis! They killed my mother and my father and my sister …' Poor, poor Samuel, and he's just one victim out of so many.

Brian grinned and said to Mum, 'Look at her face.' He turned to me again. 'What's wrong, Jean?' He began tapping with a spoon on a milk bottle. 'Come on, answer me.'

He stopped tapping. 'Mum, why isn't Jean like us?' he asked. 'Why is she so different?'

'I've told you before to stop saying that,' Mum said as she put the kettle on. 'She's not different.'

'I should bloody well hope I *am* different,' I exploded. 'It's not my fault I was born into a crackpot family.'

Dad and Brian laughed at this, but Mum was indignant. 'Don't include me in that. I'm not a crackpot,' she said.

'Neither am I,' said Brian.

'Oh yes, Brian, you are definitely a crackpot,' Mum said. 'But Jean's not a crackpot, and neither am I.'

'Hey, Jean, if you're not a crackpot, then why are you a nuthouse patient?' Brian asked. 'You can't answer that, can you?'

'Shut up, Brian. I've told you before to stop saying that as well,' Mum said. 'You've got no sense.'

'At least I'd got enough sense not to go into High Royds.'

Well, he has got a point there, I thought bitterly.

Brian grinned again, and resumed making a noise: belching, animal noises, jingling coins and tapping with a spoon on a milk bottle. Clink. Clink. Clink. Each sound jarred inside my head, my stomach churned and I felt like screaming.

I skipped tea and went up to bed.

The night wore on. I was wide awake. And aching. Aching all over. I tossed and turned until I was sweltering hot. My blankets were in a lumpy, soggy ball. And I couldn't stop thinking, thinking, thinking. Could I afford a bed-sit on my DHSS giro until I got a job? Yes, there must be a way. Other people without jobs lived in bed-sits and they didn't starve, did they? I went downstairs for the newspaper and, struggling against waves of nausea, headache and fears of impending insanity, I scanned the accommodation column and drew a circle around a few possibilities that were the cheapest.

Almost anywhere would do for a start till I got a job, till I felt better and got on my feet. God, I wished this damn headache would ease up, I couldn't think straight for it. What about hostel accommodation? Cheaper? A YWCA perhaps? And would living with other people be good for me, help me get over my shyness? Live at a hostel, get a bed-sit later. Yes, that seemed – dared I use the word? – sensible.

I took the telephone directory upstairs and sat in bed flicking through the pages. No YWCA here in Bradford, but there might be one in Leeds. I'd ring round tomorrow; yes, that's what I'd do. Got to make a start, it was now or never, my last hope. But there was nothing I could do then at three in the morning so I had to try to get some sleep. Hell, I couldn't stand this headache and my mind was racing feverishly. *Must switch off. Must get some sleep ...*

Came four in the morning and I was sitting up in bed, my mind a frothy, seething whirlpool. They had messed up my life ... Can the blind lead the blind? I was nowhere near as screwed up as this when I first saw a psychiatrist. If only I could get back to how I was then and start all over again. Without psychiatry. Without drugs. Oh, if only ... *Dear God, please don't let it be too late.*

My pillow slithered off the bed to join the blankets on the floor. I picked it up and hugged it to my chest. How had this happened? How in the name of common sense and sanity had it happened? I was a teenager ... I had a job, was coping, could think clearly. But I was sad and confused about life, wanted someone to talk to, felt I needed help. Without encouragement from anyone else and against the wishes of my mother, I asked to see a psychiatrist, and agreed to come into hospital. Naïve. Trusting. Unaware. So why, then, did Sister Oldroyd accuse me of denying I needed help? And why did she believe I was secretly not taking the drugs when she snatched at my palm?

Get undressed. You're having some more Shock Treatment...

No, no, no. I cried into my pillow.

God help you if you slip back!

Dr Prior warned me not to stop taking pills. Slip back to what? I was much better before I started on them. You *must* keep taking your tablets ... No, no. I listened to you then but I won't now, not any more. I want to live.

I was confused, disorientated, exhausted. I badly needed to sleep but something didn't make sense and I had to try to sort it out right now. My brain raced on feverishly. Then I thought I'd got it. My case notes were wrong! That was it, of course. That was why they gave me all that inappropriate treatment. It was all some kind of misunderstanding right from the beginning. A wrong diagnosis. Because they didn't know me at all.

I'll have to see Dr Shaw and tell him my case notes are wrong, I decided. Sister Speight, while reading my case notes, had once told me that Dr Sugden wrote I was quiet and

259

withdrawn in Thornville. But had he failed to record how, right up to being admitted, I was going out with friends, and that I was never quiet and withdrawn with my close friends, at least not until *after* I was heavily drugged? Perhaps Dr Sugden hadn't realised that? After all, he'd never even met me except for the two brief interviews before admission, never even seen me when not on tranquillising drugs. And then, WHAM! Hospitalisation, heavy drugs, ECT ... But it was all there in my diary – dancing at the Mecca only three days before my admission. No, they can't have known all this or else surely they wouldn't have treated me as they did. And what about Sister Oldroyd misjudging my shyness as an 'attitude' and wrongly believing that I thought everyone was against me? Had her misinterpretations of my behaviour gone down in my case notes? Did other staff, then and today, think it must be true if a member of staff had said it?

Yes, I'll have to tell them my case notes are wrong, I thought. But they won't believe me, they won't listen, they won't admit it.

But they'd have to. Other people could confirm most of these things. They'd know it was the truth if they spoke to my family, my friends, and the people I used to work with at Lee's.

The anger inside me boomeranged back and forth between being directed at psychiatry for what it had done to me, and at myself for complying. Once somebody sets foot inside one of those places, they can never get out of their clutches. My mother's warning. And I had just laughed. Laughed! Take no notice of me if you like, but one day you'll remember what I've just said, she had warned me. And you won't be laughing then.

'Oh, Mother, you were right, I'm not laughing now,' I whispered as I pressed my forehead into my pillow to mop up the perspiration. 'I'm not laughing now.'

I could understand my naivety in believing I was going into hospital for 'about a week' and for 'a rest and observation'. That's what Dr Sugden had told me, and how was I to know any different then? But even when I'd been given strong drugs from the day of admission, and ECT after barely a week, even when I was being pained and humiliated and virtually destroyed, I let them do it. And I kept on letting them do it. Who was I to think I'd more sense than my family? Even Brian had more sense than to allow that to happen to him. So when my family said things which seemed silly to me, supposing they were right after all? Like my mother's warning about psychiatry? How could I trust my own perceptions about anything? The ground was slipping away. I was light and hollow. But then I re-entered myself with a new surge of anger against psychiatry because they had let my mother be right and *she shouldn't have been right!*

The night was long and dark and perilous. Unlike the well-spaced, clear-sighted, rational insights of the previous night, my thoughts tonight were tumbling about in my head and then spilling out in a jumbled heap. A mixture, I realised, of balanced and unbalanced thinking. I thrashed about on the bed as I struggled to sift out precious insights buried like jewels near the edge of a cliff, regaining my balance each time I felt myself toppling.

With shaking hands, I began writing a letter: 'Dear Mr Jordan, I hope you won't feel annoyed at me for writing to you when you are no longer the day hospital charge nurse and therefore have no concern with my "case",' I began. 'Perhaps I should not be writing to you (for the above reason) and I'm going to try not to post this letter. If I do it's just because I feel at the end of my tether and at a loss as to who to confide in …'

I never meant to send it. The letter was just a means of getting my jumbled thoughts down on paper as if I was confiding in someone while trying to sort out my sense from my nonsense. I wrote about how I'd felt worse since the Case Discussion Meeting. I expressed my concern about how Dr Shaw, even with my case notes in front of him, didn't seem to know that I, alone, had made that decision to see a psychiatrist in the first place at a time when, despite my depression or whatever, I'd been coping, 'functioning' as they called it. I wrote, also, how it bothered me that Dr Shaw had said I'd be seeing more of him in future. I didn't feel he understood me at all.

When I finished the letter, I stared at the words. Words belonged to the world of logic and order, but I knew now there were other worlds, other truths: that some things, important things, couldn't be put into words. Still, they would have to do. Words were an inadequate but necessary tool. I tore the page from my notepad and let it join my blankets on the floor, then fell into a restless sleep.

Time to get up when I realised, with shocked surprise, that my nightgown and the sheet on which I was lying were soaking wet. Sweat? Urine? Whatever it was, it wasn't normal. Panic! Heart beating fast. *Thud, thud, thud.* Too fast, too loud. Imagination switched on to 'high'. Feverishly high. I could imagine I was turning into a quivering lump of jelly that might dissolve leaving no trace of me except my soggy nightgown and a wet patch on the sheet where I'd been lying. I held out my hands in front of me and watched them trembling. Mr Jordan had told me this tremor was a side effect of my drugs. So what was it now? I tried to control it with my mind but to no avail. And then it wasn't only my hands. I was shaking all over. I felt sick.

I dashed to the toilet and, gripping the edge of the bath for support, I thought: I'm going insane, I'm going insane … I clung to the bath, still shaking all over and sweating in fear, until somehow I managed to get a hold on myself. When the anxiety attack subsided, I filled the basin and had a good wash. I wasn't going to vomit after all and, if I was going insane, I said to myself with a wry smile, at least it was to be postponed for a while.

I felt shaky and sick again when eating toast for breakfast and my head ached horribly. So I phoned the day hospital and told Tony I wouldn't be coming in as I'd got flu. It wasn't a lie: I thought I probably had got flu.

Back upstairs, I picked up from the floor beside my bed the letter I'd written to Mr Jordan. I glanced at the untidy writing,

262

crossings out and noticed spelling mistakes but didn't bother to correct them. I put it in an envelope which, with shaking hands, I addressed, stamped and sealed. Then I went out and posted this letter which I'd never meant to send.

On my way back from the post box I went into a phone booth and, true to my resolve, dialled the number of the Leeds YWCA which I got from Directory Enquiries.

'Hello, YWCA.'

Was I strong enough to do this now that thoughts were buzzing around my head like a swarm of angry bees? Supposing I was bordering on madness, about to tip over the brink? The way I felt now made that easy to believe.

'Hello! Hello! This is the YWCA.'

Supposing I did need the drugs? Dr Prior had warned me never to stop them. Oh, Lord, supposing he was right after all?

'Can I help you?'

I couldn't speak.

I'm crumbling, I thought with horror. I can no longer think straight. I'm mad!

'Can I help you?'

Speechless, I replaced the hot, clammy receiver that kept saying, 'Can I help you? Can I help you?'

Who in the world could help me now?

CHAPTER TWENTY-TWO

A FEW DAYS AFTER giving up the pills I was sitting facing Tony across the desk, the letter I'd sent to Mr Jordan in front of him beside the ominous manila file.

'What do you want me to do with this?' he asked, pointing to the letter.

'Do what you like with it,' I said, wishing he'd at least take it off the desk out of my sight. It embarrassed me.

'I've been reading your case notes,' Tony began.

'You'd be wasting your time less if you read the *Beano*.'

'And if it's any consolation to you, there's nowhere in your case notes that says "This patient has got ..." There's no diagnosis.' He stabbed the blotting paper with his pen. 'That's lucky, you know.'

'Lucky?'

'Many patients have things written about them, a schizophrenia diagnosis, for instance, that could go against them for the rest of their lives – in terms of jobs and things.'

No diagnosis? I didn't know until many years later when I read my case notes that Dr Sugden had given me a schizophrenia label right from the start and, in the letter from Dr Armstrong referring me to the day hospital, I had been described as suffering from chronic schizophrenia. So why did Tony say this? I don't know. All I knew at that point was that I had suffered greatly during the past years, was still suffering, and that my suffering had been very much worsened by my treatment.

'Lucky? Oh yes, aren't I a lucky girl?'

Tony either didn't notice or chose to ignore the angry

sarcasm in my voice.

'Actually Dr Copeland and Mr Jordan believed your problems weren't mental illness at all, but just the normal turmoils of an intelligent teenager, and … and I'm inclined to agree with them.'

'I'm not a teenager now,' I said, unconsoled.

'Are you feeling better than when you wrote that letter?'

'I'm OK,' I said guardedly.

'Are you sleeping all right?'

'No, but I'm OK.' I was biting my fingernails and aware I could hardly manage to sit still. 'I'm OK,' I said again, trying to convince myself, as well as him.

'Are you?' Tony said, with a look that frightened me. He fingered the letter. 'Anyway, what do you want me to do with this? I could put it in the bin if you like and that would be the end of it.'

'What does it matter what I want? You'll do what you like with it anyway.'

'I'm asking *you* what you want me to do with it.'

I tried to remember what I'd written in it about Dr Shaw, aware that, unless it was binned, it would be there for Dr Shaw to read. Still, what did it matter?

'What do you want me to do with it?' Tony asked again.

I looked steadily at Tony, decided he meant well and that I liked him a lot, but felt irritable.

'Do what you like with it. Why are you going on about it? Put it in the bin, stick it on the wall, staple it to my blasted case notes or … or wipe your backside with it for all I care!' I heard myself say.

'I don't think you're quite yourself, are you?' he said quietly, his eyes watching me intently. 'You've been rather agitated for the last few days. We could prescribe some extra pills to calm you down and help you sleep.'

'Stuff the bloody pills,' I retorted, wondering why it had taken so many years for me to say that. 'I've finished with pills.'

'Jean, love, you're not making this easy for me,' Tony said,

265

brushing his forehead. 'Do you realise you're not well physically? Your blood-test result shows you're anaemic and your urine sample showed up a urinary infection. Then there's this weight loss, which is becoming very worrying.'

'Well, I will keep taking the Complan,' I conceded.

I'd been steadily losing weight for several months even though my appetite remained good. And this despite me eating bigger dinners and substituting tea or coffee at breaks with the large mugs of Complan, a nutritious milky drink the nursing staff gave me three times a day. I was down to less than 7 stone, which was definitely underweight for my height of 5 feet 5 inches. The nurses had been weighing me each week for some time, and noting the steady decrease. In the few days since coming off drugs, the rate of the weight loss had become alarmingly rapid.

Later that day Dr Baines-Bradbury, the hospital superintendent, came to the day hospital. Tony sent me to see him in one of the consulting rooms upstairs.

'Sit down, Jean. I'd just like a chat with you,' he said. The manila file was open in front of him and the letter I'd written to Mr Jordan was on top of that.

Fortunately for me, I found him approachable and was able to explain calmly how I'd like to leave home and was thinking of trying the YWCA in Leeds. He asked if I'd like him to arrange for a social worker to help me with this move. I hadn't even known there were social workers at the hospital. I hesitated. I wanted to do it myself, but remembered my abortive phone call, and my self-confidence was low, so I accepted his offer.

Finally, he asked if I felt better than when I wrote the letter to Mr Jordan.

'Yes, I do,' I replied, while taking care to keep my hands below the desk level where he couldn't see that I kept tensing them up, showing the whites of my knuckles. 'Does it seem ... Do you think I'm ...'

'I don't think you're on the brink of a serious psychotic illness,' he said, with a twinkle in his grey eyes.

'Don't you?' I said, feeling greatly relieved because during the past few days this had been my biggest fear. I'd forgotten for the moment that I'd decided not to take any notice of what a psychiatrist might think of me.

'No, not at all,' he assured me, smiling at my obvious relief. 'One day you'll look back on this, wonder what on earth all the fuss was about, and laugh.'

At last things were moving. I saw Mrs Winters, a psychiatric social worker, who rang Mrs Stroud, the warden at the YWCA in Leeds, while I was with her in her office. Apparently Mrs Stroud had some apprehension about offering me a room, but she agreed, after making it clear that the hostel could give no kind of 'after care'. Mrs Winters, a grey-haired, bespectacled woman, beamed at me after her negotiations.

'Mrs Stroud's a bit wary about accepting patients but I've persuaded her to give you a try. She says you must leave immediately if you present any problems that might distress the other residents.' She fingered the pearl necklace which hung over her grey twin-set. 'We don't need to worry about that, do we?'

'No, of course not,' I said, feeling heat rising to my cheeks.

That evening I went into Brian's bedroom to get the suitcase I'd be needing. My eyes rested on a huge pile of Denis Wheatley books on the floor. I shivered. Could people or places really become possessed by evil? And wasn't Brian a bit too interested in the occult? An eerie sensation crept through my body.

'What's up?'

I jumped. Brian was standing by the door watching me, grinning. 'I saw that look on your face just then. Don't you like me books?'

I said nothing, picked up the case and left the room.

Again, sleep didn't come easily to me that night. I was thinking about good and evil, and back on the old restless search for meaning. I tossed and turned until the morning light was streaming through my curtains and I still hadn't found any answers – for how can one possibly even begin to understand?

The following evening I was packing my case as Mrs Winters was due to call in the morning to drive me to the hostel. Brian was laughing, jingling coins and clinking with a spoon on a milk bottle. Mum was crying and telling me she'd get a lodger to have my bedroom who would be more grateful than me, her own daughter. This was a repetition of the scene when at seventeen I'd announced my intention of leaving home. Oh, if only …

I was still feeling delicate since stopping the pills, and the way my skirts swivelled round my waist reminded me I was still losing weight. I hurriedly packed my case, then decided to escape the commotion by getting out of the house for a while.

I caught a bus into town and sipped Coke in a coffee bar. I thought that if I could hold myself together for just another week or two I might be OK, but I was scared by how bad I kept feeling. Shaking, sweating, insomnia, aches and pains, and most frightening of all, difficulty in thinking clearly. Did that mean I really did need the pills I'd been swallowing in handfuls each day for the past few years? Was it a choice between a zombie-like existence or … or what? Surely I couldn't remain like this for much longer. Something was bound to happen if I stayed off the pills. Sanity or madness? In which state would I surface?

I gazed out of the window, battling with fears that I was losing my mind. I marvelled at how well I was hiding it. Here was I teetering on the precipice of the dark pit of madness but looking for all the world as if I was just another customer sitting enjoying a Coke. No doubt the other people in this coffee bar thought I was gazing out of the window thinking what other young people thought about. And what might that be? Boyfriends, pop songs, clothes, trying out a new hairstyle perhaps? Oh, it would be lovely to be wrapped up in things like that, instead of having to put all my energy into trying so hard not to fall apart.

My pride at how well I was managing to hide my unease suffered a blow when Kenny, the proprietor, tapped on my shoulder and asked if I was all right. I'd liked Kenny ever since I'd seen him go outside before he locked up one night to give a sandwich to a tramp who was leaning against the window. Glancing up, I realised the coffee bar had emptied. It was eleven o'clock and he was waiting to close.

'Yes, I'm OK,' I said quickly, standing up.

'Wait,' he said as I opened the door. 'Are you *sure* you're all right, luv?'

'Yes. Why?'

'You're as white as a sheet.'

Another night of restless thought, punctuated by snatches of fitful sleep, but in the morning I was up and ready early, waiting for Mrs Winters. Some hasty cleaning and tidying had taken place in anticipation of her visit. When she arrived, Mum bustled about in a nervous manner, handing me my suitcase and fetching my handbag. Then, after commenting that I wouldn't stay at the hostel long and would soon be back home, she burst into tears and disappeared upstairs. She just couldn't accept that her baby should grow up and leave home. (Brian was to continue living with my parents until he got married at the age of thirty-six and then he ceased all contact with his birth family).

I hurriedly buttoned my coat and left with Mrs Winters. My mother came back downstairs and stood looking through the window, her face streaked with tears, then she watched from the door. As I walked down the path with my case, Mrs Winters turned to her and said, 'She'll be back.'

CASE NO. 10826

MEMORANDUM

Ref. Miss Jean Davison   Date.   18th July 1972

From. Mrs D Winters   To   Dr E Shaw
     P.S.W. Dept.

On 12th July I called at this patient's home to escort her to the
Y.W.C.A. Hostel in Leeds. The home is a semi-detached house
which I think is owned by the Corporation. It is comfortably
furnished, with wall-to-wall carpeting, a television and a
modern gas fire, but had the rather neglected look which
houses tend to have where all the members go out to work.
Both house and garden were very untidy.

Only Mrs Davison and Jean were at home when I called and
Mrs Davison was helping Jean to get her things ready to go to
the hostel. She had very little to say, in fact was rather
distressed and said 'Of course she won't stay there – she will
be back soon', after which statement she burst into tears and
left me and went upstairs. As we left the house she was
standing in the window mopping her eyes. Because of her co-
operation in helping with preparations for Jean's departure, I
think her emotion was caused by her daughter's illness and
not by the fact that she was leaving home.

CHAPTER TWENTY-THREE

'HAVE YOU WORKED OUT your finances regarding this move?' Mrs Winters asked as she drove me to Leeds. 'Of course, your parents will have to give you some financial support.'

I didn't know what to say so I said nothing. I wasn't expecting or wanting my parents' financial support, and intended managing on my DHSS money until I got a job.

'Do you go out at nights?' she asked, changing the subject.

'Yes, but not as much as I used to,' I replied.

'Where do you go?'

'Pubs.'

'Now come on, Jean. You go to more interesting places than pubs. You go dancing at the Mecca. I happen to know that.'

Recently, a secretary at the day hospital had seen me at the Mecca. I felt like a schoolgirl who had been caught out telling lies. But I wasn't a schoolgirl and I wasn't lying. Perhaps I should have been more explicit and said 'usually pubs but sometimes we go to dances afterwards'.

'Do you go out on your own at nights?'

'No, with friends,' I said, then wondered if I should qualify this by saying 'but I did go out on my own last night to a coffee bar'.

'You've got friends? That's lovely. Have you thought of sharing a flat with a friend?'

'Yes, I'd like to do that, but my friends live with their parents and they don't want to leave home yet,' I explained. 'A girl rang me a bit since to discuss sharing her flat, but she ... Anyway, I don't fancy sharing with someone I don't know.'

'But you *must* know her if she rang you,' Mrs Winters said.

I stiffened. 'No, we've never met. She asked a friend of

mine if she knew anyone who might want to share her flat. My
friend gave her my number, so then she – this girl called Nikki
– rang me.' I paused, wondering whether to say more. 'She
seemed very much taken aback when I told her I was a patient,'
I added.

'Oh, but you're not a patient.'

'What?'

'You're not a patient.'

At first I couldn't think what Mrs Winters meant because of
course I was a patient. Then I got it.

'When I told her I was a *day* patient,' I corrected myself.

I wondered why Mrs Winters was querying everything I
said throughout the journey. Ought I to be more explicit? By
the time we reached the hostel my nerves were in shreds and I
found myself being excessively precise in reply to her
questions.

'Have you packed some soap?' she asked as we got out of
the car in a street lined with large old terraced houses.

'Yes. I mean no. Well, it's not really soap,' I stammered.
'I've got some face-cleansing lotion that lathers like soap and
some foaming body wash to use instead of soap.'

I drifted through the form-filling, the preliminary chat with
Mrs Stroud the warden, and my goodbyes to Mrs Winters. I
was thankful to be left alone in my room on the second floor. It
had a long shelf across one wall, a tall, narrow wardrobe, a
large old-fashioned chest of drawers with an oval mirror on a
stand on top, a small table beside the bed, and a gas fire with a
slot meter.

I unpacked a few things, then bolted the door and lay on the
bed. I'd hardly slept since stopping the drugs about a week ago,
but now I slid easily into an exhausted sleep. I dreamt someone
was frantically rattling and banging on a door.

'Open the door, Jean! Open it at once! Jean!'

Mrs Stroud? Her tone was frightened, urgent, insistent.
Perhaps there was a fire! I rushed to the door. Mrs Stroud
looked first at me and then past me into the room, then back at
me. 'Are you all right? What are you doing?'

'I ... I was asleep,' I mumbled apologetically.

'Well, you don't need to bolt the door. Please leave it unbolted in future.'

I nodded, feeling puzzled at the fuss. Then I remembered how Tony had told me that her initial reluctance to accommodate me at the hostel was because a previous resident, a former High Royds patient, had locked herself in her room and attempted suicide.

'I'm painting the window frames in a bedroom down the corridor. Come and watch. It's no fun sitting in there on your own, is it?'

I followed her down the corridor, knowing she meant well, although there was nothing in the world I would have liked more than to be left alone to sleep.

'The other girls are out now. A few of them have jobs but most are students. We're well situated for the college, polytechnic and the university, you see,' she explained as she stirred a pot of rich brown paint. I was sitting on the mattress of the stripped bed, screwing my eyes up in the harsh glare of the sunlight streaming from the uncurtained window. 'We've a girl living here now who was in care.' She loaded the paintbrush. 'Her name's Marianne and she's a lovely girl. I'll introduce you.'

There was silence for a while except for the swishing noise of the brush on the window frame. The overpowering smell of paint was giving me a headache, and I searched my mind for an excuse to go back to my room for some much-needed sleep.

'Marianne might be in now,' she said, putting her brush down on a wad of newspapers on the windowsill. 'Let's go see if we can find her, shall we?'

Marianne, an auburn-haired, freckled-faced girl of about sixteen, was in the lounge watching horse-jumping on TV. After introducing us, Mrs Stroud left us sitting together on the old fashioned, high-backed settee.

'Oh, look. Isn't it funny?' Marianne said, giggling and pointing to the TV. 'Just look at that horse's tail.'

I laughed, too, but wasn't sure what I was supposed to be

273

laughing at. A clip of film was repeated in slow motion a few times showing some horses jumping over fences, and each time Marianne roared with laughter, pointing gleefully at the horses' tails as they slowly swished up and down. I stayed in the lounge just long enough, I hoped, not to be impolite.

'I'd better go to my room now,' I said. 'I've a letter to write.' I stood up self-consciously. 'See ya later.'

I was lying on the bed sleeping again, dreaming about horses' tails this time, when there was a knock at my unbolted door. I sprang up at once, feeling guilty for lying there. 'Do you know your way round Leeds?' Mrs Stroud asked. I shook my head. 'Well, this street map should help you. I've put a cross to mark where this hostel is. We're about fifteen minutes walk from town. To get to the town centre you take this road...' She traced her finger on the map, but I couldn't take it in. My head felt to be stuffed with cotton wool and my eyes just wanted to close.

When she left, I spread the map out on the table and tried to work out how to get to the road where I'd be catching my bus to the hospital tomorrow. I knew the name of the road and eventually found it on the map, but couldn't work out how to get there from the cross marking the hostel. Did I turn right or left from here? The more I stared at the map, the more it looked like a maze that didn't make any sense. My mind seemed to be slowing down, switching off, blanking out. Dear God, I whispered, I'm losing my faculties. Help me.

I was about to lie down on the bed again when there was another knock at the door. 'Marianne will show you where the shops are,' Mrs Stroud said cheerily. 'The weather's lovely so the two of you might as well go for a walk. She's waiting for you in her room. Bring your map.'

Mrs Stroud led me down the corridor to Marianne's room where the three of us pored over the map. I couldn't take in anything to do with the directions and could barely make sense of ordinary conversation. Without warning even to myself, I broke down and cried. Mrs Stroud put an arm around my shoulder and led me back to my room.

'I'm OK,' I said between sobs. 'Just tired. I'd like to sleep for a while if that's all right. I won't bolt the door.'

When Mrs Stroud left me alone, I thrashed about on the bed, now unable to sleep. I was too worried about what was happening to me. And of what I feared would happen if I didn't manage to get a hold of myself.

Later that afternoon, I went out alone for a walk. It only took me a few minutes to get lost, then I spent what seemed ages wandering the streets, exhausted, trying to get my bearings. It was then that something frightening happened, which seemed to confirm my worst fears.

Turning round a corner into a cul-de-sac I saw some big white letters chalked on a wall, which said PSYCHIATRISTS ARE NUTS. I smiled to myself. What a coincidence that I should come across these words now of all times. I turned back down another street and walked along for a while. Then suddenly it hit me. Surely there had been no such words on a wall? I stopped dead and leant against some railings. 'Jesus, I'm hallucinating now!'

I don't know how long I stood there, leaning against the railings. This is the end of the line. I've gone crazy, I thought despairingly. Soon they'll take me away to a mental hospital, and I can't stop it happening. I can't alter the script after all. I've tried. I've tried so hard.

When I started walking again, my legs held me up even though they felt like paper. I felt thoroughly wretched – weak, distressed, aching, shivery and weary beyond belief. I wondered again if I'd got flu, but feared it was something far worse than that. I was curious to see if the writing was still on the wall but I couldn't remember how to get back to it. That's if there even was a wall … Hallucinations were a brand-new experience and the thought of them terrified me. How could I tell what was real if I couldn't trust what I saw with my own eyes? Was this street I was in now real? Were these houses in front of me real? Was anybody else out there real? Was I real? I pinched the flesh on my arm; something could feel it, something must be real. But what is reality when we only have our perceptions?

I continued to wander aimlessly until a telephone kiosk loomed up in front of me. I found the number of the hostel in the torn, worn directory, dialled with trembling fingers and got through to Mrs Stroud.

'I can't find my way back. I'm lost,' I said. How true of my life, I thought wryly.

'What's the name of the street you're on?'

'I don't know.'

'Doesn't it say so in the phone booth?'

'Oh yes, it's Clayton Street.'

'Well, Jean, you're only a few minutes away. Take the first turning on your left then the next on your right and ...'

It was useless. I couldn't understand the simple directions.

'Will you ring High Royds for me, please. Tell them I ... I need to be admitted because ...' I gulped back my tears and brushed aside a remaining speck of pride, 'because I'm mentally ill.'

I could hardly believe I'd just said that. If I was mentally ill, then the last place on earth I'd be safe in would be a mental hospital. I'd be safer roaming the streets and sleeping wrapped in newspapers.

I'll have to run away, I thought. But where to?

'Stay right where you are, Jean,' Mrs Stroud's disembodied voice crackled through the telephone wires. 'I'll be with you in one minute.'

A few minutes later I was in the brightly lit dining room of the hostel eating roast beef and potatoes amidst a crowd of chattering students. I was ravenously hungry although I hadn't realised that until I'd started eating. My last meal had been a small piece of toast over twelve hours ago.

After tea, I went to bed, taking care to leave my door unbolted. Mrs Stroud had said nothing about my request for her to ring the hospital to admit me. I had requested it in my most despairing moment of weakness, but wouldn't agree to it now. OK, so I might have experienced a hallucination when roaming the streets stressed, hungry, exhausted, probably physically ill.

And also (perhaps most significantly, though I lacked full awareness of this, then) while I was in the throes of a 'cold turkey' withdrawal from drugs.

I felt I was living on borrowed time. It was as if after years of remaining static, I was on the brink of getting a lot better or a lot worse. I was still sustained by the way everything had flashed so clearly in my mind when I'd realised the destructive effects of my treatment and stopped taking the pills. Why, then, I wondered, after facing myself with undiluted truth that had at last prompted me to take necessary steps for my well-being, had I become more unsteady, more emotionally strained, more psychologically vulnerable, than ever before? Was I wrong to stop the pills after all? Had I really got some kind of mental illness that had only been held in check by drugs? Why was I getting a frighteningly good vantage point of those cliffs about which Gerard Manley Hopkins wrote? I'd once bought a second-hand poetry book and knew the words by heart from some of the poems I could relate to.

> O the mind, mind has mountains; cliffs of fall
> Frightful, sheer, no-man-fathomed. Hold them cheap
> May who ne'er hung there.

As I was drifting off to sleep I heard someone crying in the next room. Her bed must be parallel with mine up against the other side of this thin wall, I thought sleepily, and she's crying in bed. I was much too tired to be kept fully awake by this but, throughout the night, I kept hearing this sobbing. Whatever was wrong with the poor girl in the next room?

In the morning, as I was getting dressed, I caught sight of my face in the oval mirror, and froze. A pale face stared back at me with very red, very swollen, eyes. I looked, and felt, as if I'd been crying for hours. All night perhaps? I gasped. That girl I'd heard crying was *me*!

CHAPTER TWENTY-FOUR

I TRIED TO HIDE with make-up the signs that I'd been crying all night in my sleep, but knew I looked awful as, self-consciously, I entered the crowded, noisy dining room. There were about seven tables, each holding eight people, and a long, narrow table at the front for cutlery, crockery, a packet of sliced bread, a dish of margarine and a toaster. After waiting my turn to use the toaster I sat at the nearest vacant place: a table with seven Chinese girls engrossed in conversation in their own language.

Many of the others had bacon and eggs with their toast, so I went through to the kitchen and found that cartons of eggs and rashers of uncooked bacon had been put out for us. A few girls were standing, laughing and chatting, around the large frying pan but, hungry though I was, the simple act of joining them to fry some bacon was too daunting. Instead, I returned to the dining room, gingerly poured some coffee from a large metal jug, and toasted another two slices of bread.

I ate my breakfast quietly amidst the clatter of cutlery and noisy chatter. When Marianne passed my table I made an effort to smile but my lips twitched nervously. I was getting the sweats and shakes again. It's no good, I thought, panic increasing my heart beat to an alarming rate. I can't make it. I can't. I breathed deeply several times: I can't but I *must*. I *must* and I WILL.

After breakfast I sat in my room, wondering what to do. I didn't want to go to the day hospital. But what might happen if I didn't show up, especially in view of my panicky phone call to Mrs Stroud last night? On no account must I agree to admission. But could they section me? Oh God, no! I washed my face again, bathed my eyes gently and then sat on the bed hoping that if I waited a while my eyes would become less puffy and I'd look less ill. It would be too dangerous to let mental health staff know how bad I was feeling. But how could I hide what showed so clearly in my face?

I looked in the mirror again. No improvement. Oh yes, here's a patient who's definitely in need of drugging and shocking. Be a good girl and drink this nice Largactil syrup. Sit still, dear, while we rub conducting jelly in your hair and clamp these electrodes on your head. Don't be a naughty girl, we're only trying to help you.

I brushed some pink blusher onto my chalk-white cheeks, blended it carefully with my fingers as it said in the magazines to try to achieve a natural healthy look, and forced a smile onto my lips. They're not going to look so closely at me, I thought. Perhaps I looked at least passable from a distance. I stood back, and stared in dismay again at the mental patient in the mirror. Oh shit! Well, it was the best I could do. I'd have to set off now. And for heaven's sake, I told myself as I fumbled to fasten my coat buttons, don't let them see how much your hands are shaking.

After getting lost and wandering around town, I toyed again with the idea of running away. It did seem a safer option than risking being admitted. Where could I go to lie low for a while, be anonymous, and keep away from psychiatrists, at least until I felt stronger? Had I enough money to get me to London or somewhere? Yes, just about. I headed for the railway station. But the prospect of trailing the streets of London cold, hungry, homeless, alone, held only slightly more appeal than returning to the hospital and saying, 'OK, you win. I'm sick. Do what you like with me.'

I sat on a bench, watching a tramp scavenging in a rubbish bin.

Hours sneaked by.

I moved on to the station buffet, ate a cheese sandwich, and then back to sit on the bench. The tramp I'd seen earlier returned. He sat down beside me, muttering unintelligibly.

More time passed. The sky darkened and spat upon us.

Finally, I returned to the hostel and ate my tea, shyly, amidst the chattering crowd, feeling isolated and alone. Then I went to bed.

Next morning I woke early, pulled on my jeans and T-shirt, and breakfasted on coffee and toast before the dining room filled. I wanted to lie on my bed all day but feared Mrs Stroud might ring the hospital to say I wasn't functioning. Perhaps I should go to the day hospital, especially after missing yesterday? But supposing the staff there decided I looked ill enough to require admission? My dilemma was the same as it had been yesterday morning: I was in no fit state to allow myself to be seen by psychiatric staff. I counted the money in my purse. Train fare to London? No, that was a crackpot idea. I went off out to find where to catch the bus to Menston.

I arrived at the day hospital, feeling desperately sad and vulnerable. The two student nurses moved on every few months. Andy, whom I liked, was working on a ward now, replaced by Clive who had been nagging at me for the last couple of weeks to wear a 'nice dress' instead of my usual jeans and T-shirt. As if what I chose to wear was any of his business.

Instead of going to OT we'd been staying at the day hospital recently to do some unpaid work called industrial therapy, which this week was packing greetings tags for a local firm.

'We've got enough packers at the moment,' Clive told me, 'so you can sit at that other table and do something else.'

I sat at the table where Maud and Ethel, two elderly patients, were sitting staring blankly while rocking back and forth, their mouths working in that constant chewing motion I'd seen in many patients. I thought these were symptoms of mental illness but learnt later they were indicative of a drug-induced disease called tardive dyskinesia – caused by the same drugs I'd been prescribed for the past few years. Last week Maud had shown me a photograph of the attractive young woman she used to be. I wondered, with a shudder, what the future held for me.

Clive placed a child's colouring book in front of me, opened at a picture of a duck, then went away to return a few minutes later with a jamjar of water and a paint box. I picked up the brush but resentment, unsuppressed by drugs, rose inside me. I was a woman who was being treated like a child. Why?

Clive was looking over my shoulder. 'Don't forget to paint its beak,' he said. 'There's some yellow paint here, look.'

Obediently I dipped my brush into the water-filled jamjar, and then into the yellow paint in the box labelled 'Children's Rainbow Paint Box'. But then something I'd once read somewhere jumped into my mind, jolting me out of my pathetic compliance: 'If they give you ruled paper, write the other way.' Clive was pointing to the beak telling me to paint that. I daubed the paint on the duck's webbed feet instead.

'There, that's the beak done,' I said when I finished painting the feet. 'I'll paint its feet now. Ducks have bright blue feet, don't they?' I began painting the beak blue while persisting in calling it the feet. Clive looked puzzled.

'But those are the feet and that is the beak,' he said, pointing them out to me.

'Oh, really?' I said in mock surprise. 'Are you certain of that? Things aren't always what they appear to be, you know.'

I continued to purposely mix up the various parts of the duck's anatomy, and the perplexed look on Clive's face made me want to laugh in spite of myself.

'You're doing this on purpose, aren't you, Jean? You *do* know the difference, don't you? You're playing games with me.'

But he didn't seem sure whether I was or not. I knew my behaviour was dangerously foolish, but I think my reasoning was along the lines that if I was about to go mad anyway, then I might as well squeeze my last bit of fun out of life first, instead of continuing to stifle myself by conforming to the wishes of the staff.

Clive took the paint brush from my hand, filled it with yellow paint and gave it back to me, telling me to finish painting the duck with that, then he went away to watch other patients. I tried to resign myself to the idea that it must somehow be my own fault; perhaps I deserved to be treated like a child to punish me for acting like one or something; perhaps I didn't understand because of my sickness that this hospital really was giving help. But as I tried to understand, anger swelled up into a big black pain inside obliterating all else. I loaded the brush with paint as black as my feelings and, in a few swift strokes, the duck disappeared in blackness.

Clive returned and looked over my shoulder at the page.

'Why have you done that?' he asked.

'Go and look in your psychiatric textbooks and see if they will help you to understand why I've done that. Then you can come back and tell me.'

Dr Shaw arrived and I was called into his office. In a rush of words before my courage failed me, I told him my case notes were wrong, my treatment was wrong, and being asked to paint pictures in a nursery child's colouring book was an insult to my intelligence.

'Of course, painting a duck is no worse than many other forms of so-called therapy,' I added. 'Like being asked to stand in the grounds shouting "Hot Peas" or jumping around saying "I am silly".'

'I've no idea what you're talking about, and I am fed up of your silly talking which has gone on for too long,' Dr Shaw told me, banging his pen on the desk, a tap to emphasise each word of 'which-has-gone-on-for-too-long'.

'You've just said you've no idea what I'm talking about. So how do you know it's silly? Why do you form opinions on things you've no idea about?'

Brave words but I was quaking inside. We faced each other across the desk like gladiators in an arena. For some reason, we always seemed to annoy each other.

'I'm not here to play games with you,' he said sternly. 'Where did you get to yesterday when you ran away?'

'I didn't run away. I'm here, aren't I?'

'Are you going back to the hostel? Or shall we admit you to Prieston Ward?'

Prieston? I'd heard that was worse than Thornville. I thought of the hostel dining room full of bright, chattering students, and felt too weak and ill to face going back there that night. I felt trapped, unsure of myself.

'Come along now. Let's have your decision,' he said, looking at his watch. 'Shall we arrange for your admission?'

Memories of my experiences in Thornville flooded my mind with pain. Never again, I resolved. Summoning up my last ounce of rebellious strength, I told Dr Shaw I would *never* go back into hospital unless I was unconscious, that I would sooner die than be admitted, that I should have learnt my lesson long ago, and, yes, of course I would go back to the hostel. I wish I could say that after this brave speech I held my head high and went back to the hostel where all ended well. Instead, I sat there close to tears, afraid of how bad I was feeling.

'Are you ill?' Dr Shaw asked. I hung my head. He could see I was unhappy, could see that he'd won. What more did he want?

'Come on, Jean, answer me,' he said, in a way that reminded me of my brother trying to rope me into some nonsensical argument. Dear God, I must be ill so why not admit it? I thought.

'Yes, I'm ill,' I replied, skulking lower in my chair and feeling painfully exhausted and defeated. 'I'm mentally ill.'

'Right then. I'll arrange for you to be admitted.'

No, no, no, a part of me was screaming. But if I'm not well enough to get back to the hostel, where will I sleep tonight? I tried to compromise.

'If I agree to being hospitalised, could it be without having any drugs or ECT?' I asked. I believed my prospects of healthy growth depended on establishing this, but it seemed a tall order if I was admitted. Dr Shaw apparently deemed this question, which was so important to me, as no more deserving of an answer than when I'd asked him if I could have a glass of water during the Case Review Meeting. He frowned and looked at his watch again.

'It's getting late,' he said, 'so stop this game-playing and make your mind up. It's back to the hostel. Or Prieston. Which is it to be?'

'I'll go back to the hostel,' I said, standing up.

Tony came over while I was putting my coat on. His lips were moving but I couldn't hear him properly; the sound kept blanking out so I was only catching snatches of a sentence, odd words here and there. I went outside feeling panicky and walked quickly down the drive. I *had* to get away or I might be lost for ever. When first admitted to Thornville, I'd been stronger and more stable than now, but still they broke me. I'd never survive experiences like that a second time, especially not in my present vulnerable state.

Although hungry, I was not sure I could face the crowded hostel dining room, so I went to the little café near the hospital where I used to go occasionally with Vera and Georgina. Aware that my money had to go far, I bought an egg sandwich, the least appetising but cheapest meal on the menu, and a cup of tea. Parts of the conversation I'd just had with Dr Shaw kept running through my mind. I'm ill, I'm mentally ill, I said to myself, feeling utterly weary and demoralised. From my table near the window I could see it had started to rain again. Didn't it do anything but rain these days?

A couple approached me at the bus stop and the man asked for directions. 'How to get to where?' I asked, trying to be helpful, but when he started repeating his question the woman tugged his sleeve and said in a voice which I did manage to hear only too well: 'Don't talk to her, David, let's go. She's one of *those* patients.' The mixture of fear and contempt on her face as she said this and pulled him away both angered and saddened me.

The bus was late, which gave me time to worry about not being able to find my way back. I felt too fragile to wander the streets looking for the hostel that night. Courage drained out of me, whatever bit was still left. I plodded towards the hospital.

On rounding the bend in the long, winding driveway and catching a glimpse of the hospital looming up large and dark ahead of me in the pale light of evening, I stopped dead in my tracks. No. No. I *won't* allow this to happen to me. If I lose this battle now, everything will be lost. I *must* get back to the hostel.

I turned and walked a few paces back down the drive, then stopped again, feeling dreadfully ill. Despite the pouring rain, I briefly, though seriously in my desperation, considered spending the night sleeping under a hedge in a field. But what about tomorrow? Where could I go? Where did I belong? I didn't feel I belonged anywhere and wished I could melt away into the ground. Pushing my fringe out of my face I tilted my head upwards to catch the cool, soothing raindrops on my hot, aching forehead. Then, feeling as if I was walking to the gallows, I trudged towards the main entrance.

I rang the 'Enquiries' bell in the foyer and said to the tall, thin-faced man, presumably a night porter, who peered through a glass partition at me: 'I'd like to be admitted to this hospital.' The look on his face almost made me smile despite my misery and fears. With widened eyes and a gaping mouth he looked completely gormless. Cautiously, he slid the window open a little further and stared through the gap at me.

'What is it you want? Who are you?'

'I'm a day patient,' I explained. 'My doctor is Dr Shaw. When I saw him earlier today he said I could be admitted and I said ... I said I didn't want to be, but ... but now I've changed my mind.'

'Dr Shaw's gone home. You'll have to come back tomorrow.'

I hadn't anticipated any difficulty in getting myself admitted for surely anyone who walked into a mental hospital like that asking to be taken in must be nuts enough to require it immediately.

'But I'm ill. I'm mentally ill,' I informed him indignantly. Surely this was the Open Sesame password. He scratched his head and stared at me.

'Oh, can't I be admitted now?' I begged him.

It was unbelievable. *This can't be happening to me, it can't. It's all just a strange dream.* How many times had I thought that during the past few years? How many times? Now here was I, after all my hard-won insights and firm convictions about the harmfulness of psychiatry, after my previous experiences as an in-patient, after all that optimism and certainty that I was right when I stopped taking the tablets and after, only a few hours earlier, telling Dr Shaw I'd sooner die than ever become an in-patient again – here was I *pleading to be let in.*

After asking my name the man at the reception window disappeared, saying he was going to try ringing Dr Shaw at home. He returned about fifteen minutes later and asked, 'Do you know where Prieston Ward is?' I nodded.

'Well, go and report to the sister on Prieston. She's been told to expect you.'

'Thank you,' I said, looking up at him and sharing his obvious relief at solving his little problem.

Thank you? The final irony! Where would it end? Perhaps next I'd be crawling on my knees before my keepers saying: Thank you for teaching me I'm sick, thank you for screwing me up, and thank you, oh thank you, for turning me into a mental patient unable to function in the outside world.

I endured the humiliation of admission procedures quietly and co-operatively. The sister, who looked not much older than me, and another young nurse, giggled at their own private jokes as they frisked me over.

'I'll have to take that from you but you'll get it back later,' Sister said, pointing to my pendant. I handed it to her and she opened it to look at the photographs inside of myself aged seventeen and Mark, one of my former boyfriends who had bought me that pendant and put our photos inside.

'Is that really you?' Sister asked.

I felt embarrassed. She might well ask if the long-haired, smiling teenager in the photograph who looked wide awake and full of life was really me. Was it? Oh to be seventeen again, even with all the confusion about life and religion and everything just the same as it was then, I thought wistfully.

286

'He's nice. Is he your boyfriend?'

'No, not now. I haven't seen him for a long time. I ... I don't know what made me wear this pendant again,' I stuttered, feeling myself blush.

'Hey, come and look at this,' she said, calling the other young nurse over.

A tired-looking doctor with an enormous stomach hanging over his trousers arrived to give me a cursory medical examination. For some reason, which no doubt made sense to him, he kept prodding and tapping the soles of my feet as I sat with my legs stretched out on a bed.

'I thought my head, not my feet, was the problem,' I said in a weak attempt at a joke, which he met with a surly look.

I was given a hospital nightgown to wear, a large, shapeless utility garment with a neckline that hung almost down to my waist. Curling up between the crisp, white sheets of the hospital bed, I fell asleep at once. But somewhere between night and day, I found myself lying in the shadows staring up at a green light, like the one I'd seen a few years ago in hospital. Hospital? Oh, please not the hospital again, I whispered. Please let it be just a bad dream that I'll wake up from soon. I closed my eyes tightly to shut it out but when I opened them again the green light was still there. I blinked, rubbed my eyes and made sure I was awake. But that green light was still there. It really *was* there.

Perhaps I'll *never* be able to get away from this place, I thought, as an icy breeze wafted over me, chilling my bones.

CASE NO. 10826

The few days she spent at the Y.W.C.A. proved to be an intolerable strain because she felt isolated and alone and could not mix with the large number of girls and young women. She finally ran away in desperation and could not face a return to the situation at the hostel.

Dr Shaw

CHAPTER TWENTY-FIVE

THERE WAS ONE FAMILIAR face in Prieston Ward: Elsie, whom I'd played draughts with on my first day at the day hospital. She was in a confused, restless state: rocking, mumbling to herself and seemed afraid, agitated.

'Hello, Elsie,' I said, sitting beside her in the day room after breakfast and gently stroking her hand. She calmed down but stared at me blankly. Then her face lit up in recognition.

'Oh, hello, Jean. Have you come to see me?'

'I've come to join you,' I replied.

A nurse pushed the drugs trolley into the room. I was given vitamin and iron pills. And Melleril. I didn't feel strong enough to attempt to refuse the Melleril and, anyway, I was unsure now that I should. Although still keen to be free from drugs, it had occurred to me that ceasing abruptly was not a wise method.

The patients in Prieston were all elderly women, except for Katie, Anita and myself. Katie, a long-haired, jeans-clad teenager, carried a denim shoulder bag covered in brightly coloured little round stickers depicting a funny smiling face and the words: 'SMILE, GOD LOVES YOU!' Anita, a wife and mother, perhaps in her late thirties, sat silently staring into space most of the time, but occasionally she would turn to me and say: 'I don't want any treatment. I've never been right since I had ECT.'

Lisa sat smiling to herself, while Hilda, a small, plump woman, kept pulling up her wrinkled stockings and saying to anyone and everyone: 'Do you want a mint?' Louise sometimes exploded with, 'Oh shut up about mints, Hilda,' but most of the time nobody took any notice of Hilda's litany. Edith kept saying, 'I shouldn't be in here.' She, too, was ignored except by Louise who responded every now and then with, 'For God's sake, Edith, stop moaning. You've as much reason as any of us to be in here.'

'No, I shouldn't be here. I shouldn't,' Edith retorted indignantly. She paused. 'I'm scared of the outside world.' If she wasn't telling us that she shouldn't be in here, she was telling us that she was scared of the outside world.

Agnes kept acting like one possessed. It was a belief of my old Pentecostal church that evil spirits can possess people and speak through them. Although on the one hand this seemed like superstitious nonsense to me, sometimes I had to wonder. Agnes was a small, shrunken, hunch-backed woman. She would sit for hours slapping her head with her hand, saying 'Damn you, God! Damn you, God! Damn you!' in a deep voice that sounded different from the pathetic voice which sometimes pleaded, 'Leave me alone, go away,' in between the curses against God and the string of obscenities that poured forth. Once, after the 'Damn you, God!' had been going on loud and long, Agnes stared across at me and 'the voice' that had just been cursing God cried out: 'It's all right for that young girl over there.' Agnes was pointing across directly at me but her eyes looked unseeing; I'd heard she was almost blind. 'It's all right for her,' the deep voice continued. 'Hers is only for a time, but ours is for eternity.'

Could it be possible that demons, jealous demons, were speaking about me, saying that my suffering was only for a time but they would be banished to hell for all eternity? Or was that a very sick way to think? I decided I'd better try to push these thoughts from my mind, along with the thoughts about psychiatry doing me harm, until I felt stronger. I would think about it all later, but I knew that now, while walking a tightrope across a dark chasm, was not the right time. All I had to do at present while Agnes was ranting and raving at me, while all around me was darkness and confusion, was to look straight ahead and concentrate on keeping my balance, retaining my sanity.

Anita asked me the way to the toilet and when I replied, 'About halfway down that corridor and it's on your right,' she waved her hand and asked hesitantly in hushed, self-conscious tones, 'Is that my right?' Later that day, while washing the mountains of crockery after dinner with several other patients, Anita picked up a damp dishcloth and began to 'dry' the plates with that, before turning to whisper to me, 'Is this a tea-towel?'

'No, this is a tea-towel,' I replied, handing her a spare one from the radiator, but my brain was so fuddled that I found myself looking at the dishcloth and thinking 'Dishcloth? For washing up?' and then at the tea-towel and thinking, 'Tea-towel? For drying? Yes, I *am* right.' And I realised how much Anita, too, was probably painfully aware of her confusion, aware that part of her mind wasn't functioning properly, scared that she didn't know where the toilet was or how to distinguish between dishcloths and tea-towels. She glanced at me with eyes that showed the humiliation of being unsure, of having to ask; the pain and fear of feeling your mind is disintegrating, your whole world is crumbling. I knew I could so easily fall from the tightrope to land on the same side as Anita but, fortunately, I managed to keep my balance.

Dr Copeland and Mr Jordan used to tell me I was different from the other patients. But now I had to ask myself, was I *really* different? I could see so much of myself in the others. In patients such as Edith saying 'I shouldn't be here'; in patients such as Anita saying she didn't want any treatment and hadn't been right since having ECT; in patients such as Katie who wanted to believe in a God who loved her. And it didn't stop there. No matter how bizarrely a patient talked or behaved, I could see in each one of them an uncanny resemblance to some facet of myself.

I was sitting among some elderly patients who might be hospitalised until they escaped in death and, seeing in them a reflection of myself, I was thinking my situation was as hopeless as theirs. But then the mirror image faded as I realised that at least one big tangible difference between them and me

291

was that they were old and I was young. My life stretched out in front of me; I might have over seventy years of it left. I wasn't ready yet to give myself up for dead.

I went across to the OT block before Sister had a chance to ask me why I wasn't there. Everyone was sitting on wooden fold-up chairs in the hall. The Head Therapist was waving her arms about at the front leading a sing-song, accompanied by another therapist playing the piano, to the sound of lots of rattling cans. Each patient was holding two cans.

'Come along now. Let's have you all singing and rattling your cans in time to the music.'

I took my place among the other patients. A therapist handed me a song sheet from the musical *The King and I* and two Pepsi cans filled with something that rattled. So there I was sitting rattling my tin cans, asking myself for the hundredth time how this could be happening to me, and singing about not letting anyone suspect that I'm afraid.

We stopped for a tea break and a tall, thin woman, who was bald except for a few wispy tufts on top of her head, rushed up and flung her arms around me.

'Jean! Oh, hello, Jean. It's so good to see you.'

I looked at her, trying in vain to recollect who she was.

'You don't recognise me, do you?' she asked, looking a little hurt. 'Oh, Jean, it's me. Georgina.'

'Georgina! But I thought …'

'You thought I'd snuffed it, didn't you? I was in a coma for ages, but here I am. Back from the grave.'

Back from the grave seemed an apt description for someone who looked more like a walking corpse than the Georgina I'd known. She pulled a chair up and brought her cup of tea over.

'The doctors didn't expect me to live,' she said. 'When I came out of the coma Dr Shaw was bending over me saying I was the luckiest person alive because I'd pulled through against the odds. Lucky? Why can't they understand that I want to die? I think people should have the right to take their own lives if they want to. Don't you think so, Jean?'

Good old Georgina was forcing my brain to creak into

292

action. A brain that could barely manage to think further than dishcloths and tea-towels was being pushed back into thinking about the deeper issues of life and death.

'Perhaps so,' I said slowly, pulling my thoughts together and trying to sort out my views. 'If I had a terminal illness that was leading to a slow, agonising death, I'd like to have the right to speed things up a bit if I chose. But don't you think when you're feeling better, you might be glad they didn't let you die? I know it's awful to feel depressed but these feelings can pass.'

Georgina looked thoughtful. She shook her head. 'If I decide I want to die, I should have the right to kill myself. Oh well, here's to another failed attempt.'

I wondered if it wasn't so much that she'd attempted to kill herself and failed, but rather that she'd decided to take all the risks but allow fate to make the ultimate decision. How much longer could she go on playing Russian roulette with her life?

My parents came to visit me. Brian brought them in his battered old Mini. I saw Brian only briefly when it was time for my parents to leave. He stood looking around the ward and I saw him watching Agnes banging her head. I thought Brian's face showed a mixture of embarrassment and curiosity. He seemed anxious to leave.

On another visit my father came alone. We sat facing each other at a Formica-topped table in the dining room where patients normally sat with their visitors. He began telling me his troubles: how Brian and Mum were getting on his nerves and so on. My expression might have made him realise that I didn't want to hear all that. He stopped. 'But I shouldn't be burdening you with *my* troubles now, should I?'

After an awkward silence he put his hand on the table and moved it along in crab-like motions. 'Look, Jean. I've brought my pet crab to see you.'

'Dad! I'm not a child any more,' I said coldly.

He looked hurt. I felt guilty, knowing he'd meant well. We sat in silence while I stared miserably at the now collapsed crab lying flat on the table.

Celia, my newest friend who I'd met through Mandy, visited before leaving for Paris with her fiancé. The following day Celia's sister, Helen, came to see me, much to my surprise. I'd only met her once before when I'd had tea at Celia's house. She was such a warm, friendly person that my shyness with her soon melted. We planned to go to a beginner's course of dancing lessons when I left the hospital. When I left the hospital ... My optimism grew. Things were going to be all right.

Mandy wrote to me. She'd just got engaged and her letter was full of happiness as she described her ring and wedding plans. She said she wanted me, her best friend, to be a bridesmaid and that I'd better hurry up and get out of hospital so I could go for my dress fitting.

'Does anyone want a mint?' piped up Hilda.

'Yes please. I'll have a mint,' said Ada, a new patient.

I broke off from reading Mandy's letter to watch as I'd been wondering before what would happen if somebody took Hilda up on her offer. Ada came over to her holding out her hand for the mint.

'You can't have one,' Hilda retorted indignantly.

The two women glared at each other, then Louise intervened.

'If you've got some mints, Hilda, then give Ada one. Have you got any or haven't you?'

'No, I haven't,' replied a subdued Hilda. Louise could be quite formidable.

'Well, why do you keep asking people if they want a mint when you haven't got any?' Louise snapped. 'You're bloody mental. No wonder you're in this place.'

I chuckled to myself, but then another little drama unfolded and this one pained me.

Lisa stood up and announced: 'Life's too short for arguing, isn't it? Let's have some fun. I'm going to make you laugh.' She danced, clowned about in front of us, told some jokes, tried to organise some party games, while all the time her eyes looked sadder than sad. She got no response from her audience except from Louise who sighed, yawned, and said, 'Oh for heaven's sake, Lisa, sit down and shut up. Can't you see you're getting on everyone's nerves?'

Lisa continued her comedy routine. Perhaps at some time in her past she'd been the life and soul of the party. Not here. She was the saddest clown I had ever seen. She tried hard to organise some games, tried to get participation from her drugged, unhappy audience, tried hard to make us laugh and it was so sad that it made me feel like crying.

It's all there in a mental hospital: life in caricature; the whole gamut of human emotions. Like Edith, I used to think 'I shouldn't be here' and, looking back, I don't suppose I should have been. But who should?

For a time, I lived with these people and my fate became entangled with theirs. But only for a time. From the shadows of a mental hospital ward, I listened and waited and watched the world – the world of Agnes, Louise, Edith, Lisa and all the other patients, of the doctors, nurses, bleak corridors, drugs and ECT. That world was painfully confused. It was dark and long and narrow, like a tunnel. But somewhere outside was a different world, bigger and wider with plenty of room for me. I decided that if it still wasn't too late, if I wasn't going to spend the rest of my life in a drugged semi-functioning state, then one day I would write a book about all this.

I leant back in my armchair in the day room and took stock of my life. Now I was back as an in-patient, this time in a 'chronic' ward where most of the other patients were old women with, seemingly, no hope. They were waiting to die. Whatever aspirations may once have flowered inside them had withered. My heart ached for them but my sympathy, like my good intentions, was no help at all to them and a threat to my own well-being. So I was trying desperately, though somewhat unsuccessfully, to be unaffected by my present surroundings, and to close my eyes and mind to the sadness of those around me.

Sometimes I seemed to be doing extremely well in this respect. I had even got to the stage where I could smile at the jokes in the book Helen had brought me, while the patient sitting next to me was saying repeatedly in a pathetic, pleading voice: 'Please God, let me die, let me die, I can't bear it, I can't go on ...'; while Agnes opposite was banging her head sharply with the palm of her hand, screaming, 'Damn you, God! Damn you, God! Damn you!'; while Edith, whose vacant, senseless expression cruelly mocked her words, was saying for the umpteenth time to anyone who cared to listen that she most certainly should not be in here, but that she was scared of the outside world.

Iris, as usual, was not saying anything but was causing the most disruption. She was a tall, well-built woman who was probably in her mid-seventies. She walked with a stoop and looked as if she was carrying the whole world on her bent shoulders. Her deeply lined, ashen face, with a permanent frown, was a pathetic picture of woe. Her eyes revealed the depths of misery and despair. I had never seen such sad eyes. She rarely said anything and spent her time plodding up and down, back and forth, pacing the ward, much to the annoyance of staff and patients alike. The nurses would shout at her to sit down and keep still, but really they were asking the impossible. She was so restless she could not sit still for more than two minutes. I think she really did try and, at times, I felt indignant at the nurses' lack of patience with her, but I tried to accept that they had a difficult job.

This day, Iris was pacing about as usual and the ward sister and another young nurse were talking about her. As psychiatric staff sometimes do, they were talking about her as if she wasn't there, or as if they assumed that she was too ill to be fully aware of what they were saying.

'She used to be a dancing teacher,' Sister was saying.

'Really?' said the other nurse. 'Well, who'd have thought that?'

'Oh yes, it's true,' continued Sister, 'and some of her pupils became well known. She was really good, you know. She won lots of medals and trophies.'

'Good heavens, she never did, did she?' said the other nurse, who seemed to me to be unbelievably naïve. Surely she didn't think that all the patients here had always been in their present state?

I glanced anxiously at Iris and I knew she was listening. She was listening and remembering. I wished the nurses would go away to the office if they were to continue this conversation.

'Hey, Iris,' the sister called to her. 'It's true, isn't it, that you used to be a dancing teacher?'

Iris didn't answer. She just kept pacing about looking utterly forlorn and dejected as the nurses continued talking.

Suddenly, she stood still and, for a moment, the expression in her eyes changed, and I thought her memory had awoken to something connected with happier times long ago. Almost at once, however, her eyes seemed to cloud over with bewilderment and confusion. She stood there as if in a trance and then she said in a flat, apathetic voice before she continued her wanderings: 'My dancing days are over.'

I thought about her dancing when she was young, happy and healthy. I thought about her being presented with those medals and trophies, which she was once, no doubt, so proud of. Where were they now? Of what use were they now? 'My dancing days are over,' she had said. I thought about those words …

… I still do.

Outside, life was going on. Outside, people would be laughing, crying, hurrying to and fro about their business or strolling in the sunshine. Babies would be crying; children would be playing; all would be living. I had been part of that world once and, 'God' willing, I would be part of it again. Most of the poor souls in this ward never would. 'I'm scared of the outside world,' Edith said over and over again. 'It frightens me.' Hadn't it once frightened me? Hadn't I once said I was more scared of living than of dying? Certainly, life outside held many problems and there was, indeed, much sadness there. But had I been so blind as to see only the sadness and not the happiness, the evil and not the good, the wrong and not the right? What a distorted vision. Now just as Edith was afraid of the outside world, I was afraid of this inside world. Surely, a sick mind, depression, could never be healed in a place such as this hospital. A place where hope is destroyed, aspirations frustrated, light and humour repressed. A place where people die and yet their bodies live.

I wandered out of the dull, stuffy ward into the bright sunshine. The contrast to the depressing atmosphere of the ward was enormous. The sky was blue with not one cloud in sight. The occasional breeze, which rustled the leaves on the trees, cooled the baking air. Overhead, the birds were chirping, and in the distance in the fields the baby lambs were playing.

I walked as far as the bench shaded by the tree near the day hospital and sat down. I still felt weak and ill physically, but inwardly I could feel a deep sense of peace, and sitting there in the bright sunlight, watching the birds fighting over their food, and feeling the gentle breeze ruffling my hair, I was aware of a sense of balance, harmony, perfection, which was far beyond the comprehension of us creatures bound by earthly restrictions.

It was a feeling to be enjoyed, not thought about and analysed. If it was merely 'a feeling' then perhaps it would burst like a bubble under the critical eye of analysis. No, I dared not dwell on what I was feeling, or even think about it at all, lest by thinking about it, it would be lost. God? Does He exist? I still did not know and, at that moment, it did not really matter. It was enough to feel that there was 'something'. In a world of many wrongs, some things were right, beautifully right. I wanted to be in this world and to take my rightful place within it. With all my heart, I wanted to live and be whole. And with so strong a desire for this, a natural healing process was able to work unhindered.

CHAPTER TWENTY-SIX

SOMETHING TREMENDOUSLY IMPORTANT HAD happened to me, something beyond the grasp of my understanding. How could I ever be the same again? But here I was, back as an in-patient, back on drugs, and feeling as fragile as a butterfly emerging from a cocoon. So where was the victory? Yet I was sure that a turning point had been reached. It was all up to me now but, having stumbled upon a reserve of inner strength and serenity, I *did* have the ability to make it. I knew I did. Be careful, Jean, I warned myself. Don't get too optimistic. Remember that old joke about the light at the end of the tunnel being the headlamps of an oncoming train.

I still saw getting off pills as a necessity but decided that next time I would cut down gradually. Meanwhile, I directed all my energy into preparing for a future in the 'outside world'. I got my parents to fetch me the shorthand textbook I'd bought years ago. Office work might be boring but I was hardly in a position to be choosy. And now that I was facing myself with clear-sighted honesty, I would delay no longer in being honest with Mike. I wrote to him in New Zealand and told him everything.

While the other patients were sitting around the TV in the evenings and weekends, I went into the Quiet Room with my shorthand book and set about the task of forcing my brain to work. I had to start from the beginning even though I'd supposedly been learning shorthand at OT for quite some time. As when I'd been a schoolgirl trying to do my homework, there were certainly distractions to learning here. One such distraction came in the form of a tall, slim young woman called

Annabel.

Annabel wore an immaculate bright red trouser-suit with black patent leather high-heeled shoes and a crisp white blouse with a ruffed neckline and a black bow at the front. Her fair hair was cropped short and fell in a fringe over her pale face. The bright red lipstick she wore, which matched her suit, did not detract from her blue eyes, which gleamed with intense brightness. She paced about while keeping up a constant monologue as she acted out her personal dramas, often reaching a frightening pitch of aggression with threatening words and gestures.

'This is a brothel! Why have they taken me to a brothel? I will not remain here. Mother! Fetch my coat at once. I wish to go home immediately. Do you hear me? And you, young lady, with your oh-so-saccharine smile, *you* are the owner of this brothel!'

When Annabel wandered into the Quiet Room where I sat alone with my shorthand book I tried to ignore her and carry on learning.

'Did you hear what I said?' Annabel shrieked.

I looked up to find her advancing towards me waving her arms. She stopped only inches away from me and launched into a flood of hysterical verbal abuse. Her anger crackled and flared while I braced myself in the heat ready for her to fly at me as Rosie had done at OT. But it seemed Annabel's aggression was only verbal. Her eyes were fixed not on me – she was probably unaware of my presence – but slightly to my right as if she were talking to someone else. A tirade of angry words bounced around the little room that was inappropriately called a 'quiet' room, as she pointed and shouted at imaginary people.

'You! And you! Stop laughing at me. I do not belong in this den of iniquity, I tell you. I've been tricked. Where is my coat?'

I looked back down at the shorthand book and began checking the exercise I'd just completed with the answers at the back of the book. If I could learn in this environment,

300

perhaps I could stop worrying that ECT and drugs had damaged my brain?

'You're a whore! That's what you are! A whore!'

I was getting the hang of it but there were just certain phrases and vowel positions I needed more practice with before I could move on to the next chapter.

'I hate you! You're a whore!'

'Annabel, come here for your injection,' a nurse called, popping her head round the door. It took two nurses to lead the distraught Annabel away. This gave me time to practise a few more phrases before she returned to continue her argument with the owner of the brothel who was now cowering on the floor behind me.

When a thick airmail envelope with a New Zealand stamp arrived for me at the hospital, I tore at the flap impatiently, eager to learn Mike's reaction to my 'secret life'. It was a long, caring letter in which Mike expressed great surprise to hear I was a patient and that I'd been receiving psychiatric treatment for all the time he'd known me. It didn't alter his feelings for me, he wrote, since he knew me well enough to know I wasn't 'mad'. He wished I'd felt able to tell him before but said that it must have been very difficult for me to write that letter and he'd been moved to tears at how painfully honest and open with him I was now.

After reading Mike's letter a second time I slowly folded it, enjoying the crinkly feel of flimsy airmail paper, and replaced it in the envelope. Declining Hilda's offer of a mint, I leant back in my armchair in the day room to think about my relationship with Mike. I had never felt I loved him, but then what did I know about 'love' when a large part of my emotions had been dampened down for so long? I had so much to learn and relearn that it seemed almost like learning to live again.

My thoughts were interrupted by the little old lady known to us as 'Gran' nudging me and whispering, 'You see that woman over there?' She was pointing to Hilda. 'She pinches things from my locker. She's wearing my knickers today.' I couldn't help chuckling to myself at the thought of Hilda, a very fat woman, trying to squeeze into a pair of knickers belonging to the thin, frail Gran.

'I don't think she is,' I whispered back.

My weight was still causing concern. I was down to about six and half stones and my clothes hung loosely over my thin frame. But around this time, my weight stabilised and then steadily began to increase.

What to do? Where to next? I didn't want to live with my parents and I didn't want to live at the hostel. Nor, of course, did I want to linger in the hospital. But I'd been in Prieston for about a month before I managed to make my decision. I would go back to living with my parents – at least for a while. It was far from ideal, but I thought perhaps I should consider myself fortunate to have this option. It seemed that many people were remaining in hospital because they had nowhere else to live.

I asked Sister when I could be discharged. 'Today, if you like,' was her casual reply. 'But where will you live?'

'With my parents for now.'

'OK. I'll have a word with the doctor when he does his rounds,' she said, scribbling a note to remind herself. Later that morning, without further ado, I was discharged – back to living with my parents and attending the day hospital.

Back at home no mention was made of my time away. I might just as well have returned home from a shopping trip. Nothing had changed. Mum and Dad went to bingo that evening. Brian stood behind me jingling the coins in his pocket. It jarred on my nerves but I flicked through the pages of a magazine and pretended I couldn't care less.

I went to bed early and lay in the half-light, pondering over those three words of Mrs Winters that had sent shivers through me when I'd been leaving for the hostel. *She'll be back*. Had she meant back to visit my mother? Or had it been, as it seemed to me, a tactless remark in anticipation of my failure? Tears of frustration dampened my pillow while I said to myself, OK, what now? Where do I go to next? I meant where to with my life, but there was no satisfactory answer to that. Stuck again. It seemed the only place I was going was back to the day hospital. Tomorrow.

On my first day back at the day hospital I sat in the armchair next to Arnold who immediately made the effort to turn and speak to me.

'Are you feeling better now, Jean?' His words came out laboured but clear.

'Yes, thank you, Arnold.'

'Good. I am pleased.'

Arnold, who spent his time sitting mutely staring into space. Arnold, who had great difficulty in speech and movement. Arnold, who had more reason for despair than I had ever known, had remembered my name, noticed my absence and shown concern for my welfare. Dear Arnold.

After the Prieston episode I was still keen to get off medication. I wanted a life. Dr Shaw refused to agree to, or even discuss, my request for a reduction, with a view to coming off. 'But you've tried doing without medication,' he had pointed out. 'And you couldn't cope.'

The way I saw it, Dr Shaw's attitude gave me no option other than to reduce the pills myself in secret. At the day hospital we were given our tablets in small plastic containers each lunchtime, just enough to tide us over until the following day, with extra on Fridays for the weekend. We were entrusted to take them ourselves; no one there snatched at my hand as in Thornville. But before I'd started my intended reduction, an extra pill kept appearing with my supply. Thinking the student nurse was miscounting I'd meant to discreetly (not wanting to get her into trouble) mention it to her. But before I did so, Dr Shaw called me into his office.

'How many tablets are you taking?' he asked.

That was easy. I knew by heart what I was supposed to take and when to take them. I'd decided I would start reducing them soon by missing out the morning one first. But at the moment there was no need for me to lie. I was taking them exactly as prescribed.

'We know you're not taking them properly,' Dr Shaw said.

'What?'

He leant back in his chair, looking smug. 'Don't think you're fooling us.'

'Look, I know I told you a bit back that I want to stop taking them because they make me feel dull and drowsy,' I said, 'but you strongly advised that I continue with them, and that's what I'm doing.'

'Well, we have reason to believe you're not.'

'What reason?' I asked.

He didn't answer.

I left his office feeling puzzled. Later that day, I asked to speak to Tony, the charge nurse.

'Dr Shaw accused me of not taking my tablets,' I said.

'And are you taking them?'

'Yes, I am. Why does he think I'm not?'

Tony smiled. 'Can you think of any reason why he thinks that?'

'Well, I did tell him a while ago that I want to stop. Is that why he thinks it?'

Tony's smile was irritating me. He knew something.

'OK, I'll tell you,' Tony said. 'The staff have been instructed to slip an extra tablet into one of your containers now and then.'

'Whatever for?'

'To test you. It seems you hadn't noticed, so Dr Shaw thinks that shows you've been tipping them out instead of taking them properly.'

So that was it? How ridiculous, I thought.

'I *did* notice.'

'You didn't say anything.'

'No, I didn't, did I? Silly me for not thinking the staff would be playing some kind of stupid game to test me.'

Tony laughed.

'It's not funny,' I said. 'No wonder patients get paranoid.'

I thought afterwards about the way Sister Oldroyd had clutched at my hands thinking I wasn't taking my tablets. And now this. The staff's attitudes also showed in their words 'compliance' and 'non-compliance'. It didn't seem right to me. If we wanted to reduce or stop our medication, why on earth couldn't we have the opportunity to discuss it, be given honest information, and our decisions be respected?

I began to reduce my pills. As my body gradually adjusted to taking fewer drugs, some of the drowsiness lifted and I was able to take more interest in things. But one of the nurses used me as an example of the need to persevere with drugs. This was when Lizzie complained that her new tablets were making her feel awful and drowsy.

'But look at Jean,' the nurse said. 'She used to complain of being too drowsy on her tablets but now she's adjusted to them and she feels a lot better. So just keep taking them and after a while you'll be much better, too. That's right, isn't it, Jean?'

Lizzie looked at me with questions in her eyes. I winced, averted my eyes and said nothing. I had given up hoping I could get the day hospital staff to understand that it was right and important for me to reject my treatment, so I just wanted to lie low and get myself off the drugs with as little hassle as possible. But I felt terribly guilty for betraying Lizzie with my silence.

Several more months passed, during which time I'd been slowly reducing my pills, before I expressed my desire to try living at the hostel again. I squirmed in my chair in Mrs Winters's office while she telephoned Mrs Stroud to try to get her to agree to me returning to the YWCA.

It was 1973. Precious time was slipping by and I still hadn't secured a job or accommodation. My heart leapt when I heard Mrs Stroud at the other end of the phone finally say, 'Oh, all right then, we'll give it another try. After all, we are supposed to be a Christian organisation.'

Mrs Winters put the phone down and smiled. My relief at

being offered a room helped me relax enough to make a jokey comment. Mrs Winters threw her head back and laughed. 'Oh, Jean!' she exclaimed, her eyes wide with wonder. 'You're almost normal!'

She looked pleased with me. Perhaps she thought calling me 'almost' normal was giving me a compliment, upping my self-esteem? I stared down at the carpet, retreating back into my shy mode.

At home that evening I began packing, while trying to ignore my mother's negative comments and tears. I kept telling myself that I was doing the right thing. But behind my brave front lurked the fear of winding up in Prieston as before.

CHAPTER TWENTY-SEVEN

I WAS GIVEN AN attic room with a sloping ceiling. It contained most of the things I needed and some things I didn't, such as the dead cockroach I found beneath the bed and the cheeky mouse which I awoke to find sharing my pillow. The window was too high to see through unless I stood on a chair which wobbled precariously as I stretched up, gripping the windowsill, to either gaze down at chimney pots and grey slate rooftops or up at the sky.

Occasionally, during my first couple of weeks at the hostel, hysterical laughter rang out in the middle of the night from the room next to mine, which housed a woman whom the other residents called 'Nutty Norah'. She gave me such a fright one night when I awoke to find her standing in my room, though I guessed she had innocently wandered there after going to the toilet. 'I'm so sorry,' she said, and fled. They put us mad ones up in the attic as in *Jane Eyre,* I thought, smiling to myself.

There was a gas fire in my room and a hungry meter which was forever running out of money. How quickly the room would turn cold. Orange, glowing flames shrank to white apparitions, flickering and dancing to that annoying popping sound – *phut, phut, phut* – as I searched for the appropriate coin. I hadn't much money but my parents did help by giving me 'money for your meter' which they saved for me in little polythene bags. (My mother had soon forgiven me for being so ungrateful a daughter as to leave home.)

Shyness was still a major problem. At mealtimes if anyone spoke to me or if I tried to join in conversation, I could hardly swallow, the cutlery shook in my hands, my heart hammered and I felt hot and sticky: all those old, familiar feelings that froze me into silence. After the evening meal I either retreated to my room in defeat or ventured into the communal TV lounge, only to find that once inside I could do no more than sit quietly among the chattering crowd. Would I ever belong anywhere? But I remained optimistic about building up a life for myself, though I knew it would take time. I wasn't expecting a rose garden.

The next stage towards leaving the hospital had to be getting a job. I applied for a clerical post with the Civil Service, passed the written examination and was called back for an interview. It began to go badly when I tried to answer, with scrupulous honesty, the questions of the man and woman who were interviewing me. This meant explaining about my lengthy period of unemployment. The man in particular seemed extremely embarrassed at my revelation that I was a day patient at High Royds, His pale face flushed crimson and he shuffled about in his seat. After a silence, he cleared his throat. 'I ... I won't prolong this interview,' he said, straightening his tie. 'I don't believe in, er ... in prolonging things because ... because prolonging an interview only makes things get rather embarrassing. I mean embarrassing for both parties.'

I knew before he managed to stutter out, 'We'll let you know' that I had no chance of getting the job.

I recounted the interview to Len, the new charge nurse.

'Never mind, Jean,' he said. 'You did well to pass the written test and to attend the interview.'

'How will I ever get a job? What am I supposed to write on application forms?' I'd received two application forms in the post that morning for low-level office jobs and, on each, I was supposed to give 'full details' of my 'previous employment' and 'explain any gaps'. Shit! If only I could cancel the last five years of my life and start anew. Pretend I was five years younger or something. 'What am I supposed to do?' I said again, realising for the first time the immensity of the problem. 'It's as bad as having a criminal record. Nobody'll ever want to employ me.'

'We'll see what we can sort out for you,' Len said.

A Disablement Resettlement Officer who liaised with the hospital made arrangements for me to attend an Industrial Rehabilitation Unit in Leeds. But there was a waiting list.

I sat next to a woman called Vivian in the YWCA dining room, and she invited me for a coffee. Her room looked cosy in the glow of the gas fire but I realised, with a pang of remembered pain, it was the same room in which I'd cried through the night.

It did look different though. On the small table beside the bed sat a portable typewriter with a half-typed sheet of paper inside. Piles of plain and typewritten sheets, along with an electric kettle and an over-stuffed ashtray, cluttered the floor. The oval mirror on top of the chest of drawers vied for space in between two metal filing trays and several wallet folders. A large box-file and a ring-binder occupied part of the bed. Two half-open drawers revealed more papers and binders. The long shelf across one side of the room housed a row of books.

'These are my friends,' Vivian said, pointing to the books.

Vivian picked up the kettle and, while she padded barefoot down the corridor to fill it in the bathroom, I sat on her bed and glanced at her friends on the shelf. They had names such as *The Bell Jar, Wide Sargasso Sea, The Razor's Edge, A Room of One's Own, The Four-Gated City* ...

Vivian sat cross-legged on the bed, propping herself up with the pillow. In her long blue dressing-gown and usual dark glasses she looked fortyish, much older than the other residents.

'Are you a student?' she asked, lighting a cigarette.

'No. I'm a patient at a psychiatric day hospital,' I said boldly, then in somewhat cowardly fashion added, 'but please don't tell anyone here. Only Mrs Stroud knows.'

'I've been in a mental hospital,' Vivian said. 'A long time ago.' She handed me a sheet of paper. 'This is the synopsis for the novel I'm currently working on. The theme is alienation.'

The synopsis outlined the story of Catherine, a young woman who married a Nigerian law student and went to live in

309

Nigeria. Marital problems relating to the culture clash proved insurmountable and Catherine returned to England with their two daughters. The couple divorced, and Catherine underwent a traumatic identity crisis, which led to a suicide attempt and admission to a mental hospital.

'Yes, it's autobiographical,' Vivian said as if in answer to my thoughts. She pulled open a drawer and showed me a photo of a distinguished-looking black man in ceremonial robes. 'My ex-husband. He's a barrister in Nigeria.' Another photo depicted two smiling young women. 'My daughters. They live in London.'

Hours later I cleaned my teeth in the communal washroom with the big old-fashioned sink and antiquated bath. In my attic room, I undressed, swallowed a Melleril and got into bed. By now I had cut the pills down to amitriptyline 25 mg twice a day, and Melleril 25mg at night. The Infirmary was close to the hostel and I drifted to sleep listening to ambulance sirens and thinking about Vivian, suicide, alienation. Vivian and I shared 'outsider' feelings. Perhaps that's what drew us together.

In the autumn of 1973, I had reached the top of the waiting list for the Industrial Rehabilitation Unit. At last I was leaving High Royds. But first there was something I had to do.

I wandered around those miles of corridors in the rambling hospital until I came to a sign for 'Paley Ward' where I'd heard Mr Jordan now worked. I went in and was met by a stench of urine and the distressing sight of women whose bodies had outlived their minds. They were sitting or wandering around, some silent, others muttering or wailing, while a radio was blaring out some irrelevant pop song that was currently in the charts.

Mr Jordan emerged from an office wearing a white coat and looking tired.

'Hello,' I said shyly. 'I'm leaving the hospital today, so I've come to say goodbye, and thank you.'

Leaving his sad charges under the eye of another nurse, Mr Jordan motioned for me to follow him to a quieter place at the far side of the ward where we could sit and talk.

'I'm glad to hear you're leaving,' he said. 'May I say – and I mean this in the nicest possible way – I hope you never come back.'

'I won't,' I said, smiling. 'I certainly won't.'

'How's things with your family?'

'I told my dad I had to get away from the hospital or I'd end up like a vegetable. My brother mocked me for saying "vegetable". And Dad dragged me to the window and made me look at our neighbour's cabbage patch. He said, "Those things there in the ground are vegetables. People can't be vegetables, so stop talking silly."'

I looked at Mr Jordan who had tilted his head back and was puffing clouds of smoke into the air. I'd recalled the same incident to Mrs Winters and she'd said that most non-medical people wouldn't say 'vegetable' in that context. So was it me?

'It's awful,' I said, suddenly feeling very sorry for myself. 'When I'm with my family I've got to rephrase whatever comes into my mind before I say it. Or they accuse me of "clevering" by using what they call big words. But I'm not trying to be clever or special. I just want to be ordinary, whatever that means.'

Mr Jordan sighed. 'There's one simple solution to all your problems and it's staring you right in the face,' he said, lighting another cigarette and puffing furiously.

'What?'

'Leave home.'

'Oh, I'd forgotten you wouldn't know. I'm living at the YWCA until I get a job and then I'll be flat-hunting.'

Mr Jordan looked interested, but we were interrupted by a patient with a tall, slender body bent forward and arms flailing like a windmill. She'd been gradually inching her way nearer till I could feel a fan-like breeze on my face from her arms wafting the air. A fraction nearer and I'd have to move to prevent being hit.

'Go away, Monica,' Mr Jordan said.

She backed away a little but was soon advancing again.

311

'Monica, I've told you to go away,' Mr Jordan said with mock severity in his voice. 'Go on. Push off.'

Monica moved away and watched us from a distance, uttering low wailing sounds.

'She's jealous because I'm talking to you,' Mr Jordan explained.

'There's not much to live for like that,' I observed sadly, my thoughts returning to God and my 'why?' questions.

'Like Monica? She'll be dead in less than three months. Now, what were you saying? You've left home. That's good. You'll be all right now.'

'It's not quite so simple. I can't mix with the others at the hostel because of my shyness. I am trying but ... but it's hard.'

'Sure it's hard. So what? Life's hard.'

'I keep feeling sorry for myself,' I admitted. 'But I know that a lot of people are much worse off than me.' How could I not know? Here, of all places, there were always plenty of reminders. Monica had returned to stand in front of us again, her arms still cutting the air in large circular movements. 'I'd better go now. I just wanted to say goodbye and to thank you for the time you spent talking to me at the day hospital.'

We stood up and shook hands, ducking away from Monica's flailing arms. I turned as I was leaving and saw Mr Jordan affectionately place his arm around Monica's shoulder. He seemed tired, angry, cynical, and had chain-smoked while we'd talked. He had a difficult job and he was no saint. But he was a good nurse. He cared.

I walked back to the day hospital where Georgina, a day-patient again, threw her arms round my neck and wept.

'Oh, Jean, I am pleased for you that you're leaving, but I'll miss you so much,' she said between tears. 'Don't forget about us, will you? But then it's selfish of me to say that because you're young and it's only right that you should go away and forget all about us and this awful place.'

'No, Georgina. I won't forget.'

'You will, Jean. You'll forget about us, but I suppose that's how it should be. Goodbye, Jean. I'll miss you.'

'I'll miss you, too. And I won't forget. Goodbye, Georgina. Take care, won't you, and please try to be kinder to yourself.'

I lingered for a while holding this child-woman who was clinging tightly to me as her body convulsed with sobs. After that, there were more goodbyes to say to other patients, handshakes with the staff, together with polite smiles, cheery 'all the bests'. And then it was time for me to go.

Time for me to go! Five years after agreeing to spend 'about a week' in hospital for a 'rest and observation'; five years after my initiation into the mental hospital world of drugs, ECT, humiliation and pain; five rotten, lousy, wasted years too late, and it was time for me to go.

Outside a cloudy sky was brightening. I strode down the drive resolutely looking forward all the time, while daring to hope that each new step was taking me on towards a brighter future in which the strange, sad, hospital world would be left far behind me. Goodbye High Royds Hospital. Goodbye at last. Goodbye for ever.

PART FOUR

BLESS THIS MESS

Be not disturbed at being misunderstood.
Be disturbed rather at not being understanding.

Old Chinese Proverb

CHAPTER TWENTY-EIGHT

ON MY FIRST DAY at the Industrial Rehabilitation Unit I palled up with Jenny, my age, who was fighting agoraphobia. She and a friendly young man called Gerry became my special friends at the unit. Gerry often got on the same bus as me and one morning, after getting off the bus together, he told me he was 'gay'. Not realising his sensitivity about this, I acknowledged it only briefly. Minutes later I had to stop him stepping absent-mindedly into a busy road.

'Do you know what I mean by "gay"?' he asked, still looking preoccupied.

'Yes, of course. You're homosexual.'

'Doesn't that bother you?'

'Why should it?' I asked. Did he think that because I was shy and quiet I must also be easily shocked or naïve?

I realised later, from the responses of some of the others at the unit, that I was, indeed, naïve. I'd had no idea of the extent of prejudice that still existed.

'But I am right to tell people, aren't I, Jean? I know I am,' Gerry said. 'If people can't understand, that's their problem. It doesn't bother me. I don't care what anyone thinks or says. I don't care at all.'

'It's hard not to care,' I said.

'Yeah, I reckon it is,' he admitted.

With Gerry and Jenny's help, I got talking to many of the others at the unit. Rob, eighteen and the size of a primary-school child, became aggressive when people treated him like the child he looked to be, but his strong sense of humour was never far beneath the surface. John had problems finding employment because of his prison record. Vincent was disabled through a stroke so needed to change his employment. Colin had lost two fingers in an accident, Chris had lost his hand, Bert's arm had been amputated ... Always someone worse off.

I sat packing envelopes with Karen, a blonde, baby-faced twenty-five-year-old. She told me her problems started in her teens. That was when she began 'doing drugs', got drunk every night, became pregnant, had an abortion and tried to kill herself.

Dennis Sloane, the staff instructor in charge of our section, told me Karen was immature and he felt her prognosis was poor. But I noticed how Karen acknowledged responsibility for her life, blaming only herself for messing it up. There were lessons to be learnt from them all as we each strove in our own way to overcome various obstacles.

I wanted to forget about the hospital. But my not-too-distant past was still breathing heavily down my neck and reappeared on my doorstep just before teatime one day in the form of Mrs Winters, the psychiatric social worker from High Royds.

I sat uneasily on my bed next to Mrs Winters, aware that her eyes were flitting around the room till they came to rest on the carpet.

'How often do you clean your carpet?' she asked.

'Once a week but the old, manual sweepers here sometimes pick up dirt in one place and put it down in another,' I explained.

Then Mrs Winters looked at the window high up on the wall. 'I think you should clean your window,' she said.

'That dirt won't come off. It must be on the outside and I can't get to it,' I replied, feeling hot.

'There's a club near here for people like you,' she said.

I took it she had changed the subject and wasn't talking about a club for people who didn't keep their windows clean. She fumbled in her handbag and pulled out a notebook. 'Ah, yes, this is it. The Felix Club for ex-psychiatric patients. It's on

Wednesday evenings. I could arrange for a worker to take you.'

'Thanks but … but I'm really too busy at the moment.'

'Busy?'

'Yes. I go out with friends in Bradford regularly, and I often go to Jenny's house – she's a girl I got to know at the Rehabilitation Unit who lives in Halifax. When I do stay in, I've got Vivian to talk to who lives here.'

'Really? That's lovely. And you tell me you're shy! What do you and Vivian talk about?'

'Oh, just things generally,' I said, unsure of how to reply. I'd talked with Vivian into the night about religion, politics, education, literature, writing, psychiatry, philosophy, ethics, alienation, relationships, sex, social-class differences, prejudices, inequality, feminism … the list was endless.

'Well, I'm glad you've made a friend here,' Mrs Winters said. 'I know it must be difficult for you when most of the other residents are students.'

'It's not that. It's shyness that stops me adding my opinions to the discussions at mealtimes,' I confided.

'Do you have opinions when you hear things being discussed?' she asked, sounding so surprised at the thought of it that I felt instantly deflated.

Just then the tea bell rang. Mrs Winters came downstairs with me. 'Let me know if you change your mind about going to the Felix Club,' she said, pausing at the door. 'And do ring High Royds when your pills are getting low and we'll get a community nurse to bring you some more. Are you listening, Jean?' I was glancing self-consciously around to see if anyone else was listening. Let only the uninitiated optimistically proclaim that there is no longer a stigma attached to mental illness.

Mrs Winters's visit unsettled me. I told Vivian about it later that evening.

'It's not the way *she* behaves that upsets me so much as the way *I* behave,' I explained. 'I get all shy and tongue-tied so that I can hardly say a word or make eye contact. I'm like that with Mrs Stroud and everyone else here except for you.'

319

'Yes, I know. You don't do yourself justice,' Vivian said, looking thoughtful. 'Force yourself to get over this shyness, Jean. Jump in at the deep end. Enrol for evening classes in public speaking.'

'I don't know about public speaking,' I said, 'but I'll give the idea of going to evening classes more thought.'

'Great. I'll call in at the Adult Education Centre down the road when I'm passing and see if I can get hold of a prospectus for you. The spring classes will be starting soon.'

One Saturday, when I was twelve, I went to the swimming baths alone to deal with my fear of diving. I stood at the side of the pool in my new sea-green swimsuit, my toes curled over the edge and my stomach a quivering mass of jelly. The thought of hurtling head-first into the glittering water terrified me. I looked into the bottom of the pool, took a deep breath and forced myself to do it, then immediately climbed out and plunged in again. And again. And again. I did some stinging 'belly flops', got the awful chlorinated water in my eyes, ears and nose, which made me cough and splutter, but didn't stop until I'd achieved my target of ten. When I went to buy my chocolate bar reward, I still hated diving. But I hadn't allowed fear to defeat me. And I survived.

I enrolled for a ten-week course at evening classes in 'The Art of Self-Expression'. I stood at the front and gave a talk, did some drama, joined in class discussions with help from the tutor: 'You haven't said anything yet, Jean. What do you think about this?' I went every week until I'd achieved my target of ten classes. When the course finished, I was still painfully shy. But I hadn't allowed fear to defeat me. And I survived.

Not only did I survive the classes but there was much about them that I enjoyed. Someone gave an interesting talk about the Brontë family. Some of the things Vivian and I had talked about arose in class discussions. Without being patronising, Mrs Broadhurst, the tutor, was full of praise for me. 'You've got a wonderful mind,' she said one evening. 'Always questioning, always reasoning and always able to see the other side.'

Mrs Broadhurst, a short middle-aged lady with rich chestnut hair piled neatly up on top, involved me from the start by asking me to be the class secretary. This entailed maintenance of the register, where I saw in the 'Occupation' column that I was the only one unemployed: the others were professionals. I became aware, for the first time, of my strongly working-class way of speaking, and realised how some people (had the psychiatrists?) might feel 'distanced' from me by 'me owts, nowts and summats'. Would the doctors have viewed me differently as a teenage girl expressing existential concerns if I'd come from a family and educational background where such philosophical questioning was not unexpected?

Jenny was well spoken, elegant and articulate. Her good A levels seemed to impress Mr Atkins, the DRO (Disablement Resettlement Officer) at the unit. He always interviewed us together but most of the time only discussed Jenny's career prospects while I sat next to her feeling redundant. Jenny was offered a job, with good promotion prospects, in the office *at* the Rehabilitation Unit. An interview for a clerk/typist was arranged for me with Mrs Dunn, the personnel officer at the head office of Ravens Superstores.

I arrived to see Mrs Dunn and was amazed to realise that she was rather nervous about interviewing me at first. But soon we were laughing and joking together. She asked me to start work on Monday. 'This interview hasn't been at all like I expected,' she admitted. 'To be honest, I was *dreading* interviewing you. I thought they were sending someone very withdrawn and that it would be hard for me to get a word out of you.'

I'd signed a form at the unit prior to my interview with Mrs Dunn, giving permission for my 'medical details' to be divulged to potential employers (which seems ironic now since I'd never had them divulged to me). Apparently it was these psychiatric opinions that had initially given her some pre-conceived negative ideas about me.

321

By the end of my first week at Ravens I was bored with the work, and also sadly aware of being the only person in the large, packed canteen who ate alone every day. But I was determined to retain the financial independence I had at last achieved. My employers were happy with me. I was supposed to be 'on trial' for the first few weeks under a system whereby the unit would give me an allowance instead of Ravens paying my wage, but after the first week, Ravens were happy to employ me in the usual way. They also paid for me to do a crash course of Teeline shorthand, allowing me day release twice a week for this. Jenny told me that Mr Atkins had phoned Ravens to enquire about me and they had told him they wished he'd send more like me!

I told Mrs Broadhurst, my self-expression tutor, that I'd got a job as a typist. Earlier I'd confided in her that I'd been an unemployed psychiatric patient for several years, so I expected an 'I'm pleased for you' reaction. But her face fell and she said, 'Oh!' in a tone of voice as if she'd been given some bad news. 'Do you like it?' she asked.

'I find it boring,' I admitted, with eyes cast down, feeling terribly guilty for finding it boring.

'Yes, of course. You would do. What a pity that nobody at the Rehabilitation Unit realised you've got abilities far higher than most people.'

Abilities far higher than most people? It seemed people tended to perceive me either as incredibly dim or almost a genius. No doubt the truth lay somewhere in between.

After secretly cutting down my drugs significantly before leaving the day hospital, I had become complacent about completing withdrawal. It was Mrs Winters who inadvertently gave me the push I needed to finish with pills and make a complete break from the hospital. The wheels were set in motion on the afternoon when Martin Potts, my boss and Office Manager, was out and I answered the phone on his desk at the front of the office.

'No, I'm sorry. Mr Potts isn't in at the moment. Can I take a message?' I asked, pen poised.

'Well, I did want to speak to him,' the female caller said hesitantly.

'He'll be in tomorrow morning.' I averted my eyes from Darren, the office junior, who was pulling faces at me. He was going through a phase when he thought it a huge joke to try to make people laugh when dealing with phone calls.

'Well, perhaps you can help me. My name's Mrs Winters and I'm a social worker. I'm ringing about Jean Davison ...'

I gasped. She could have been saying this to Darren or anyone. I didn't want my colleagues wondering why I had a social worker.

'It's ... it's Jean who's speaking,' I stammered, my efficient business-like tone instantly disappearing.

For a moment, Mrs Winters sounded more embarrassed than I was.

'Jean? Oh good heavens, is that really you?' She gave a nervous laugh. 'Well, here am I thinking I'm talking to the Head of the Department and I'm talking to you!' There was an uncomfortable pause. 'Anyway, it's you I really want to speak to,' she said. 'How are you?'

'OK.'

'Do you need any more tablets?'

'No.'

'Well, do let us know when you need them, won't you?'

'Yes.'

I was trying to make it sound to Darren and the other staff within earshot like I was dealing with the usual business call.

'You *are* taking your tablets, aren't you? That's important.'

I felt like asking her if she thought I would die or go stark raving bonkers without them, but I meekly replied, 'Yes.'

'Well, I won't keep you from your work any longer. I just wanted to make sure you're all right and have enough tablets.'

'Thank you for calling. Goodbye.'

That evening, in the early spring of 1974, I wrote a polite goodbye letter to Mrs Winters. I thanked her for her concern and explained that I now felt the time had come for me to finish my connections with the hospital and to stop taking tablets.

Back came Mrs Winters's reply by return of post:

I am concerned about your intention to cease taking tablets. I am sure they help to keep you well. You could get them from your GP instead of the hospital if you prefer that. If you haven't yet registered with a GP you must do so. I'll be in Leeds on Thursday and I will call at the hostel to see you ...

I flung the letter down on the bed. If enduring the awful, zombie-like state which ensued when I followed the advice of mental health professionals meant being 'well' then no wonder we couldn't communicate: we didn't even speak the same language.

I grabbed a sheet of notepaper while my feelings were still running high. 'Dear Mrs Winters,' I wrote:

I thought I had made it quite clear in my previous letter that I wish to <u>FINISH MY CONNECTIONS</u> with the hospital. However, you can come to see me on Thursday if you like as it may be better to say goodbye to you in person instead of just through a letter ...

Before sealing the envelope, I reread what I'd written and double underlined 'FINISH MY CONNECTIONS'.

The next day I registered with a GP in Leeds so that I wouldn't end up without pills before completing my withdrawal. I gave Dr Cawthorne the drugs' names from the containers and told him I'd been on psychiatric drugs for about five years. I explained how it had all begun with my need to talk to someone about, among other things, my confusion over religion. Dr Cawthorne told me he was a Christian. We talked about religion for a while, then he suddenly announced that he wouldn't prescribe medication for me. I stared at him in surprise. I'd certainly had no trouble getting pills before.

'Shall I come back for them when you've received my medical details from the psychiatrist?' I asked, convinced that Dr Shaw's recommendations would change his mind.

'I don't believe you need medication,' he said, standing up to signal the consultation was over. Then he did something that seemed odd for a doctor. He followed me through his full waiting room and outside where he stood talking to me on the gravel path. 'Come back and see me if you want to talk about religion or anything,' he said, 'but I feel I ought not to prescribe you these drugs.'

Two extremes. Both dangerous. Dr Cawthorne didn't know me but he had quickly decided I should stop medication at once (without even knowing I'd already reduced it). The psychiatrist I first saw when I was eighteen didn't know me but was quick to decide I should start medication. And no one had ever bothered to inform me of either the risks in taking the drugs or the risks in stopping them abruptly.

I arrived home from work on Thursday wondering what Mrs Winters would say about my curt letter. Mrs Stroud met me in the hall and asked me to come into her living room.

'Mrs Winters was here earlier,' she said. 'I told her you were fine. That's right, isn't it?'

'Yes,' I said, wondering where this was leading.

'Well, she hadn't time to wait. She just wanted to pass on her good wishes and she left these for you.' Mrs Stroud handed me a bunch of daffodils. A goodbye present?

I went up to my room feeling touched by this little act of kindness. I placed the daffodils in a Cola bottle retrieved from my bin, and stood them on my bedside table. I love daffodils. Up they come each year pushing their golden heads through the dark soil, bearing silent witness that winter has turned into spring. I bent forward to inhale their clean, fresh fragrance. Mrs Winters had only been doing what *she* believed was best for me. But now I must do what *I* believed was best for me (although faster than intended, thanks to Dr Cawthorne).

Over the next few days I stopped taking all medication. It

was done now. I awaited my fate.

I awoke at four in the morning after a restless night and flung back the dishevelled bedcovers. Three more hours before my alarm would ring for work. Sitting on the edge of the bed, feeling a bit delicate, I picked up my few remaining pills. I would probably have flushed them down the toilet had I not been made cautious by my previous attempt at withdrawal.

I am sure? Keep you well?

NO!

I replaced the tablets in the drawer without taking one. Standing on the chair I pulled back the curtain to gaze at the sky. The words of Mrs Winters's letter went round my head. Words which epitomised my treatment over the years and fostered psychological dependence on drugs. 'I am concerned about your intention to cease taking tablets. I am sure they help to keep you well.'

What made them 'sure'? The training, the textbooks, the theories? Certainly not knowledge of me. I stretched up and opened the window wide. A soothing breeze wafted over my face and body as I stood there in my nightgown, listening to the dawn chorus. Feeling more settled, I went back to bed and slept.

When I awoke again there was still no green light. Just radiant sunbeams flooding my room. A glowing reminder that spring, my favourite season, was here in all its glory, drenching with warmth and colour and beauty a cold, grey winter world.

CHAPTER TWENTY-NINE

NO MORE PILLS. NO more zombie days. In the spring of 1974 I really did make it. I could see, feel, taste, smell, laugh and cry. Had I ever *really* been alive before? When you emerge from a long, dark tunnel, the light dazzles.

With each passing day, my fears that something awful might be about to happen to me decreased until the psychological dependence on drugs caused by years of brainwashing, culminating in that Job's comforter letter of warning from my social worker, melted away. Out with the pills went the horrible, drowsy depression that had been a part of my life for so long. Thank God no one forced me to continue with medication. Could they have done that if today's Community Treatment Orders had been set up? I didn't fall through the net: I scrambled out of it. At last.

No more drugs meant release from a grim bondage, freeing me to start catching up on the living I'd been missing. I took driving lessons, planned a holiday with Helen, read novels, poems and non-fiction books. Intellectual curiosity awakened in me, which led me to library books on all kinds of subjects, opening up a whole new world. Vivian lent me her books, too, and our talks in her room continued to provide the intellectual stimulation that I'd never had in my life before.

My feelings about psychiatry still needed dealing with, but I had so much living to catch up on. Coming to terms could wait. I went to weekly dancing classes with Helen as we'd planned when she'd visited me in Prieston Ward. When the course finished we were still lousy dancers, but had become good friends.

Summer was incredibly short that year. It came and passed with wings. On holiday in Somerset with Helen, the sun shone for two glorious weeks and we enjoyed long, leisurely walks in the beautiful countryside surrounding Minehead. At nights I slipped into a restful sleep and, in the mornings, waking up to the sun streaming through the pink curtains of our little guesthouse bedroom, I felt good.

In September I enrolled at evening classes for GCE O levels in English Language and English Literature. My doubts about whether I had the ability for this were soon eased by the high marks I got for my work. The literature tutor said I ought to be doing A, not O levels and asked to borrow my work to use as examples to help students who were struggling. Despite this, I was still beset with the fear that ECT and drugs had damaged my brain. I could write essays which impressed my tutors and in many ways my memory seemed amazingly good. Incidents of the past few years kept returning to me in vivid detail even before I read my diary extracts which confirmed their accuracy. But my memory for faces was very poor. When characters in films made their second and subsequent appearance I often couldn't recognise them. I also kept getting lost in the college corridors, unable to remember the way to my classroom or the way out. And when talking to people (including my old friends whom I wasn't shy with) I often forgot what I was about to say. Had I been like this before the drugs and ECT? I couldn't remember.

One lunchtime I visited the large medical bookshop near where I worked and browsed through the Psychiatry section. I learnt that many of the drugs I'd been prescribed from first being admitted to hospital were 'neuroleptic' drugs, usually prescribed for 'psychotic illnesses, mainly schizophrenia'. Listed among the 'common side effects' of neuroleptics were drowsiness, lack of interest, social withdrawal, lethargy, depression: the same 'symptoms of illness' which had caused me so much suffering during the years of taking them and which had miraculously disappeared when I finally got off them. The serious risks in taking these drugs, it said, had to be weighed against the severity of the patient's illness.

What illness? Among the symptoms described for 'psychotic' illnesses, there was nothing I could relate to my experiences (though if I'd looked harder I might have come across the 'negative' symptoms of schizophrenia which, ironically, are the same as those 'common side effects' of the drugs used to treat it). I had perceived depression as my predominant 'symptom' but judging by the cocktail of drugs I'd been on – tranquillisers, antidepressants and neuroleptics – it seemed they'd been treating me for anxiety, depression, and even psychosis. Everything!

And what risks? I turned the page and read how neuroleptic drugs can cause akathasia (restlessness), cognitive deterioration, pseudo-Parkinson's disease (tremors), and tardive dyskinesia, a brain-crippling disease characterised by uncontrollable movements of face and limbs. I read that taking other types of psychiatric drugs with neuroleptics increases risk, and that patients on long-term treatment (defined as over three years) are particularly prone to developing neurological disease such as tardive dyskinesia (TD). It went on to say that risk of TD was increased further if, instead of lowering the dosage or ceasing neuroleptic medication, patients were prescribed procyclidine (as I had been) to mask the effects. Once this devastating condition takes hold, it can prove irreversible after discontinuation of the drugs that caused it. I shuddered. Fortunately, for me, I'd been fine since coming off medication. But the psychiatric profession had seen fit to put me at such risk. Why?

I glanced at my watch. It was time to go back to work but I remained sitting on the floor in the bookstore with a pile of psychiatric textbooks at my side and a sick feeling in my stomach. Having learnt as much as I could take for now about the drugs I turned to the index and looked up ECT. 'Electro-convulsive therapy (ECT) is used to treat severely depressed patients who have not responded to other methods of treatment.' Really? It seemed that much controversy surrounded ECT and the question of whether or not it caused permanent brain damage. Memory impairment was indicated as the most common side effect, 'which may be permanent'.

Questions, questions, questions again, bouncing around in a mind which was now, at long last, unclouded with drugs. Why had I been treated with such dangerous drugs and ECT? Why had these been the first, not the last, resort? Why had no one informed me of the risks? And what on earth had my diagnosis been? Surely Tony wouldn't have lied to me when he said I'd never been given one. But, then, why administer such deeply distressing and damaging treatments without knowing what they were treating?

I looked at my watch again. Damn it, I'd be late for work if I didn't hurry. I replaced the books on the shelf and returned to work still feeling sick inside. I had so many questions, so much anger, to face. I needed to think about it and sort things out. But the pain of thinking about it made me want to forget.

'The O level exams are really just like memory tests,' my tutor said, so I thought if I passed with good grades it might help reduce my worries about treatment-induced brain damage affecting my memory. I read and reread *King Henry the Fourth, Part One*, the first Shakespeare play I'd read, spending my lunchtime each day studying in the library. I had to prove to myself that my rusty, bruised brain was capable of functioning properly, that the damage was not permanent. And I couldn't allow any painful thoughts and feelings to intrude and hinder my progress.

For several months I relegated thoughts about my hospital years to the back of my mind. Then, one evening at my literature class we were reading from Harper Lee's novel, *To Kill a Mockingbird*, when I was struck by the words:

Atticus said that Jem was trying hard to forget something, but what he was really doing was storing it away for a while, until enough time passed. Then he would be able to think about it and sort things out. When he was able to think about it, Jem would be himself again.

And I thought, Oh yes, that's like me and psychiatry. I will be able to think about it and sort things out. Some day.

The first stage of that 'some day' arrived (of all times) on the eve of my literature exam (but I still got my grade 'A') and maybe it wasn't so much a case of becoming 'able' to think about it as becoming unable to push it from my mind any longer. I was tidying up my room and singing to a pop song on the radio which had topped the charts around the time of my first spell in hospital. One moment I was singing happily, then suddenly my mind was flooded with distressing feelings, which formed into a huge question mark about my tunnel years. All the pain. All the wasted time. NEED IT HAVE BEEN SO?

I broke down and wept bitterly for my lost years.

After the outlet of tears, I began writing about the previous night when I'd slept at my parents' house after going out with Helen:

Journal

As I walked down the dark street towards my parents' house, I was puzzled by several flashes of light, but when I saw Brian, with his camera equipment, I knew the explanation. Flashing lights in my face is just one of the many ways in which my brother tries to irritate me. He was looking out of the window, grinning.

'I do that at night,' he said. 'From my bedroom window I can flash a light into the window of the flat opposite. I bet that man who lives in the flat wonders what's happening when his room suddenly lights up.'

'What pleasure do you get from that?' I asked.

'Oh, I get a lot of pleasure from it,' he replied. 'I've done it at half-past three in the morning and then his light's gone on so it's woke him up, but he doesn't know what it is, then I've waited until his light's gone off and, after a while, I've done it again and then his light's gone on again.'

'But why?' I asked, although I knew it was useless to try

to reason with him.

'Why shouldn't I? We lived here before him,' he said, as if this justified his behaviour. 'Besides, I used to do that when the flat was empty, so he's not going to stop me now.'

I sighed, and looked to my father for support, but he just laughed, and went up to bed.

Brian followed me into the kitchen pointing his camera at me. The kettle seemed to take an age to boil. 'Why aren't you talking, Jean? Come on, answer me.' I ignored him. 'Come on. Don't you know it's ignorant to ignore people?' I still said nothing. He picked up a metal spoon and began banging it on a milk bottle as he often does and it makes a horrible noise.

'Brian, be quiet. I've got a headache,' said my mother, putting her hands to her head.

He continued and Mum snatched the spoon off him but Brian picked up another and the same process was repeated. He laughed idiotically. 'You can't beat me,' he said. 'No one can.' He began tapping on the table. Tap. Tap. Tap. On and on and on it went.

I often wonder how my family situation would seem to an outside observer, if he or she could somehow listen in on it all. What would be 'normal' feelings and reactions to my situation if I must (according to my psychiatric treatment) assume that mine are not?

'I still say ...' he began again. He was talking about things too daft or offensive to listen to and asking if I agreed.

I said nothing at first, but could not stop the churning feeling in the pit of my stomach.

'Don't talk so silly,' I said, despite my intentions to keep quiet. He was slinging insults at me about anything he could think of. Somehow he got round to calling me a slut.

'Shut up, Brian,' my mother said.

'Oh, balls!' he shouted. 'I'll say what I want. Look,

Jean's still not saying owt so it must be true.'

*'You talk like you're sick. You want seeing to,' I said
quietly as I poured my tea.*

*The words were out now. It was too late to regret having
said them. Now, I knew what would follow. But I would
NOT be sensitive about it. I often think that the
unhappiness inside my brother which makes him as he is
must be far greater than any depth of unhappiness I have
ever known and, I must admit, I would not wish to swap
places with him for the world.*

'I don't want seeing to. There's nothing wrong with me.
*I haven't been on a funny farm ...' Now he was really on
a sore point of mine, and so much for my good
intentions, I'm afraid. I still have not learnt to cope with
hospital memories without feeling so hurt inside, so
confused and so bitter. What happened to me all seems
so wrong, pointless, senseless and* so bloody unfair.
*Emotional wounds are very slow to heal. I sometimes get
the feeling that long, long after I come to terms with the
things which led up to me seeking psychiatric 'help' I'll
still be struggling to come to terms with my so-called
treatment and some of the things which I saw and
experienced at the hospital.*

No. Oh, no. I will *sort it all out and come to terms with it
in some way. I* will *learn to get it all in the right
perspective. I will* not *let this bitterness and confusion I
feel about it take hold of me and poison my life.*

*Brian followed me upstairs. 'What about that woman
who was walking backwards and forwards all the time?'
He meant Iris, the poor soul. 'And what about that other
one who kept banging her head with her hands? Did you
see her? Look, banging her head like this all the time.'
Brian was so impossible.*

*'Well, what about them?' I said irritably as I slammed
my bedroom door. 'What about them?'*

*I lay on the bed and stared up at the ceiling. Outside the
door Brian was making his 'animal noises'. I closed my*

eyes, suddenly feeling very tired. Yes, what about them?
I thought. What about them? What about all mental
hospital patients? And what about the terrible
misunderstandings, lack of knowledge and poor
communication between staff and patients, leading to
treatment and attitudes which can, surely, only do more
harm than good? Can nothing, absolutely nothing, be
done to help?
'Won't you do something about it, please, God, oh
please?' I prayed to the four walls and ceiling. Well, did
I really expect an answer?

It was a mistake to ring Dad from work. I should have used the
pay phone at the hostel, but I'd only intended a quick call to
arrange a visit.

'Tell me when I see you,' I said as he began telling me his
troubles: about the situation at home, even about his confusion
over religious beliefs. I explained that I couldn't listen now as I
was at work. Apparently he wanted a sounding board and he
wouldn't stop.

'Sorry, Dad, but I can't listen to all that just now,' I said
again as he continued. 'I'm at work. I have to go. This is not
the time or place.'

'Not the time or space?' he said mishearing me.

'Time or place.'

'Time or space?' he said again. 'You do say some funny
things.' He began laughing. Laughing and laughing. I pressed
the phone close to my ear and glanced anxiously at my
colleagues.

'I've got to go now,' I said, but the hysterical laughter went
on and on, then I realised it had turned to tears. Lord, what was
wrong with him? I couldn't hang up now, but was aware that
Martin, the Office Manager, would be ready for me to take
dictation.

'Dad, what's wrong?'

No reply. Nothing but the sound of hysterical sobbing at the
other end of the line.

'I've got to go now,' I said again, but I couldn't bring myself to put the phone down until the sobbing stopped. Silence.

'Dad? Are you still there? What's wrong?'

'Sorry about that, Jean. I got a bit carried away, didn't I? I must be depressed.'

'I know, but I really can't talk now. Listen, we'll talk later. I'll see you tonight. OK? Bye.'

Before knocking on the door of Martin's office with my shorthand pad, I paused to gather my thoughts: even though I love you very much and wish I could help you, I … I want you to leave me alone now, Dad. Let me breathe. Let me live. Let me be free. Please.

I simply *must* do something about my shyness, I said to myself as I sat in my attic room poring over my *How to Overcome Shyness* book. Vivian, who sometimes seemed as frustrated as I was by my shyness, said I wasn't trying hard enough to overcome it. I was trying as hard as I possibly could.

I sat quietly and self-consciously in the lounge one evening while the others there, mainly young students, chatted. I was glad when Elspeth came in. I suspected the younger ones might think me strange for not talking but that Elspeth, being older, would be more likely to understand. They were all talking about another resident and agreeing that 'if she smiled, her face would crack'. The girl they were talking about was suffering from depression, as they well knew, and had recently attempted suicide for reasons they did not know. I was surprised and disappointed when Elspeth, a teacher, joined in with their unkind remarks.

I was about to go up to my room when Elspeth said, 'And I don't like that girl who has the room on the top floor either. She never bothers to speak.'

I froze. Did she mean me? She must do. I was the only person who had a room on the top floor since 'Nutty Norah' had left a few months ago. Did she realise I was here now? She must do. I wasn't invisible. I looked down at the magazine on my lap and pretended to be engrossed in it, while Elspeth continued.

'And it's not as if she can't help it. Last Friday I saw her laughing and talking with that friend of hers who comes to see her. Oh yes, she can talk all right when she wants and to whom she wants.'

I said nothing. What was there to say anyway? It took more courage to leave the lounge than it had done to enter it. I pretended to read a while longer, then, without looking at anyone, I stood up, walked past them all and climbed the stairs to my room.

Sooty, one of the warden's cats, was sitting near the top of the stairs. I sat next to her. 'Oh, Sooty, what can I do? How can I make myself talk to people? Why didn't I at least stick up for myself just then?' The cat climbed onto my lap and I cuddled the bundle of soft, warm fur. 'I've heard them say they don't like you either, Sooty. They say you hiss and scratch whenever people try to touch you. But you're not doing that now, are you?' Deep, contented purrs were rumbling from the cat as I tickled behind her ears and stroked her body.

'They say you're a funny, unfriendly cat who doesn't like people and won't let anyone near,' I whispered as a few teardrops dripped onto her shiny black fur. 'But we know that isn't true, don't we Sooty? It just isn't true.'

CASE NO. 10826

Mrs Green, O.T. Dept., described her behaviour, admitted that she had attended the typing school over a period of two years and during that time her mental state had remained unchanged. She is still aloof, cold, isolated and impossible to know well.

Dr Shaw

(Extract from Psychological Report)

There does seem to be some discrepancies, between what Jean sees as the problem, and how she actually is. In the Day Hospital she does not appear to be as shy and introverted as she described, and at home she does have at least one friend who visits her, and with whom she goes dancing.

Also on the 16 P.F. – the profile presented is certainly not that of an extremely introverted individual and the 2nd order factor of introversion falls within the normal range. Neither does she appear to be extremely submissive – in fact the reverse appears to be true, in that she appears to be a rather independent-minded and assertive individual, in some instances. In line with this she appears to be somewhat mistrusting and doubtful about the motives of others and tends to have a rather worldly, shrewd and unsentimental approach to life.

Laura Barnes
Clinical Psychologist

I agree with her own assessment of her problem 'I find it difficult to talk to people.'

Dr Copeland

CHAPTER THIRTY

'SAMARITANS. CAN I HELP you?'

'I don't know. I'm not suicidal. Do you only deal with people who are suicidal?'

'Oh no, we're here to listen to anyone, suicidal or not. My name's Richard. Would you like to tell me yours?'

'Jean.' I had meant to use only my middle name, Margaret, but somehow couldn't bring myself to do this.

Some achievement ... After at last FINISHING MY CONNECTIONS with the hospital and getting myself off drugs, wasn't I spoiling things by giving in to this need to talk to someone? I was annoyed with myself for ringing the Samaritans.

'I'm annoyed with myself for ringing you,' I said as I watched a tramp shuffling around outside my kiosk. 'I'm OK really. It sounds nothing, but ... Oh! Just a minute.' A whiskery face was pressed up against the door. I was about two hundred yards from the hostel in a dark, lonely street near a crypt for down-and-outs. The tramp gave me a blank look, took a swig from a bottle and then turned away to pick something up that caught his eye on the pavement.

I said far more than I meant to say to Richard. I told him how I lived at the YWCA, worked at Ravens, which was my first job after years of being a psychiatric patient, how I felt so much better since stopping taking pills, but that I just couldn't overcome shyness. It was the shyness that had prompted me to ring the Samaritans. I felt I was dealing positively myself with all other problems, but this was the most unyielding.

'Why don't you make another appointment with a

psychiatrist?' he suggested.

'Because finishing with the hospital and stopping the pills is the sanest thing I've done in ages,' I said with feeling.

'But perhaps this time you could get a *good* psychiatrist ...'

His views about psychiatry, I realised, were as naïve as mine used to be before I'd had any experience of it.

I need a bloody psychiatrist about as much as I need roasting alive, I thought bitterly. 'I don't need one,' I said.

'OK. I've another suggestion. There's a club for people who have difficulties in mixing socially –'

'I suppose it's called the Felix Club,' I said with a sigh.

'That's right. Have you been to it?'

'No, but my social worker, I mean my ex-social worker, told me about it, and I don't think ...'

The tramp I'd seen earlier pulled open the door. I recoiled as the smell of his foul breath and dirty meths-stained clothing filled the kiosk. 'Gimme a cig,' he drooled. Memories of bleak hospital corridors flooded back.

'I haven't got one,' I said.

'Well, gimme a light,' he said, holding out a cigarette stub that looked long past being smokable. The stench of meths was unmistakable. God, he'll ignite if he lights up now, I thought.

'I haven't got a light.'

'Fuck off!' he said, before shuffling off down the street again. I watched him, wondering what problems I'd got compared with some people.

'What's happening? Are you OK?' the concerned voice at the other end of the telephone was asking.

'Yes, but I'd better go. It's dark and lonely in this street.'

'Please ring again, won't you? I'll be here alternate Tuesday evenings, but do ring whenever you want. Any time at all. You can even ring us in the middle of the night if you need to talk.'

I thought the owner of the middle-class voice at the other end of the phone must live in a different world from one where ringing someone in the middle of the night would mean walking dark, lonely streets to search for a public telephone that worked.

Two weeks later I rang again and Richard invited me to meet him at the Samaritan Centre. I rang the bell of a large old house nervously. A dark-haired man of about thirty, wearing jeans and a green polo-neck sweater, answered the door and, in the well-spoken voice I'd heard on the phone, introduced himself as Richard. I followed him up some stairs to a small, carpeted room furnished with four easy chairs and a low coffee table. A long-haired, bearded young man appeared with coffee and a plate of biscuits, then left us alone. We talked for about an hour. He suggested I come to the Centre every fortnight for a chat with him.

As soon as I got back to my room after the second of these fortnightly visits, I scribbled away furiously in the thick, ruled exercise book I was using as my 'Coming to Terms' journal. I don't remember where I read the words that I wrote on the front, but I understand a similar version of this prayer is commonly attributed to Reinhold Niebuhr: 'Give me the courage to fight for what can be remedied, the patience to bear with fortitude what cannot be taken away, and the wisdom to know the difference.'

Journal
I liked Richard from the beginning because I felt he was kind and warm and very sincere, but even from that first phone call some of his views and attitudes stirred up feelings of hurt and anger in me. Perhaps it's me being too sensitive about a certain subject, but tonight he had hardly settled himself down in the chair opposite me before he managed to find exactly the right words to make me see RED.
'Have you had any depressions or elations since I last saw you?' he asked.
Depressions. Elations. The psychiatric jargon for abnormal mood swings. Doesn't he know he is hurting me when he talks like that? Why doesn't he know?
I decided I would have to think about it later when alone so that my anger wouldn't be diagnosed as a symptom of

illness. I smiled sweetly at him while I raged inside. I begin talking to him about trivial things, surprising myself by the calmness of my voice. Inside I was hopping mad.

I stopped writing here, put my pen down and read what I'd written. No, you mustn't stop here, Jean, I told myself. Stay with it now and think it through. OK, so I knew my anger wasn't really against Richard. He was a catalyst helping my anger to surface. I picked up my pen again and scribbled away feverishly:

I am sick and tired and weary of almost everything I think, say or do being analysed for signs of illness. Can't I be happy, sad, laugh, cry or do anything without being 'ill'? Will I ever again be able to convince others – or myself – that I am just an 'ordinary', 'normal' person? Will the scars never heal? When I was eighteen years old I made the biggest mistake of my life. Will I have to go on paying for it for ever?

For years I was told I was sick, it was implied I was sick, I was treated as sick. And I came to believe I was sick. I meekly submitted while they moulded me into the sick role of their own creation. I let them dope me with pills and shoot electric currents into my brain. How naïve, how stupefied with pills or how damn SICK I must have been to let them add to my problems by subjecting me to needless suffering, mental and physical abuse and great humiliation. For all those years, I let them turn me into a zombie and virtually destroy me while I looked on passively through the drugged haze with hardly a murmur.

But now I want answers to the questions burning inside me. It was these same angry questions which finally broke through my drug-induced apathy and shocked me back into life, despite all the brainwashing I'd undergone. Perhaps without the angry questions

*pounding my brain I would never have found the
courage to discard all the pills which they would have
me believe I need to help keep me well.*

*Why shouldn't I be allowed to reach down and touch my
painful innermost feelings and accept them as a real part
of myself, not a 'sick' part from which I ought to be
separated? When sadness and despair are narrowly
interpreted as 'symptoms of illness' it's easy to miss the
indication that some things in a person's life need urgent
attention by facing up to, altering or accepting. All
psychiatry did for me was push my real hurts deeper
down while I was being treated in a way which might
have caused permanent physical and psychological
damage. God knows that what I endured at the hands of
the professionals was truly out of all proportion to the
unhappiness (or 'sickness' if I'm supposed to call it that)
which originally prompted me to seek their help at the
age of eighteen. And I want to know WHY.*

*Why am I sick? In what way am I sick? Won't somebody
please tell me? Is it 'sick' to feel frustrated when shyness
hides my personality and strengthens my chains? Is it
'sick' to yearn for a meaningful life, something more
than a superficial existence? Was it really 'sick' to feel
out of step when caught up in a way of life that purveyed
cheap thrills, phoney values and shallow relationships
among the psychedelic lights and tinsel-decked thorns
(Teensville of the Swinging Sixties)? Or perhaps it's all
just because as a teenager I wanted to be understood,
needed someone to talk to, and was foolish enough to try
to discuss my feelings with a psychiatrist instead of
keeping them to myself???*

*Oh, please won't somebody tell me why I have been
labelled as 'sick'? Is it because jobs like putting screws
into television parts on a factory assembly line bore me
silly and drive me to distraction? Is it because I cannot
squeeze myself into a hole which is the wrong shape for
me? Is it because I am different from my family? Or is it*

because I cry and ache and hurt deep down inside???

During my first few visits to the Samaritans, the subject of the Felix Club arose again, this time with the suggestion that I go as a voluntary worker. Curiosity finally got the better of me. Helen called unexpectedly as I was setting off, so she came with me.

A tall, thin man in jeans and trainers took Helen and me aside on our arrival. 'My name's Ernest Wormald and I'm a social worker. First, let me say it's important to understand there's no difference here between workers and members. No one is in charge.' Having said this, he took us back into the main room where he proceeded to take charge.

We sat in fold-up chairs in a semi-circle around Mr Wormald, who tried to organise a discussion but some members kept making disruptive comments. The man sitting next to Helen was constantly masturbating and I was aware of her discomfort. I remembered a little room at the OT department which bore the name 'Group Therapy'. I thought of how Mrs Winters had described the Felix Club as being for 'people like you'. And I thought perhaps I should know better now than to draw up divisions between 'them' and 'me'. But, still, I couldn't help thinking that these people had problems which were quite different from mine.

We didn't go to the Felix Club again. I couldn't see what I could offer the others there, and I certainly didn't feel the club had anything to offer me. Months afterwards Helen still kept saying, 'Do you remember that awful club we went to? Oh, wasn't it disturbing and depressing?'

Richard introduced me to Jim, the Tuesday evening leader at the Samaritans. He was a kind, caring person, probably in his late fifties, who, like Richard, spent a lot of time with me during my fortnightly visits, which were to continue for about a year. Richard soon stopped seeing me as a potential candidate for further psychiatry, so I, in turn, stopped being defensive with him. And Jim, dear Jim, never seemed to view me in that light from the start. He said I was the right kind of person to be a Samaritan and even suggested I join them.

I grew very fond of Jim and Richard. We chatted informally, laughed a lot, and built up a relationship based on trust, warmth and respect for one another. They talked to me as if they simply believed I was a perfectly normal and likeable young woman. Call it 'non-directive counselling' or 'befriending' or whatever, it was a wonderfully positive experience, not only for me but for each of us, I believe. When I decided the time had come to break contact, I knew what Jim meant when he wrote me a letter in which he said he felt I knew, too, that the three of us had been part of 'something a bit special'.

I also received a lovely letter from Mrs Broadhurst, the self-expression tutor, who said she was writing to commend me for my courage and attitude in dealing with my problems, which had, she wrote, been a tremendous source of strength and inspiration to her.

But things went from bad to worse at the hostel. It got to the stage where other girls shouted unkind remarks through my door at night. A rumour had got round that I was a lesbian, for apparently no other reason than that on Friday evenings when Helen visited me we sometimes spent the evening in my room. This, coupled with the way 'she keeps herself to herself' had made them add two and two together and get five. There was no truth in the rumour but even if I had been a lesbian – so what?

One evening as I arrived back at the hostel, two giggling girls who lived there jostled and teased me at the door. Lydia linked my arm and said to the other: 'I've fallen out with you, Fiona. Jean is *my* friend. You didn't know I was one of *them*, did you?' And then to me, 'Come along, darling. How about my place tonight?'

A few other residents who were watching laughed as Lydia tagged on to my arm and snuggled up to me.

'See you tomorrow, my love,' she called, noisily blowing a kiss as I pulled free and climbed the stairs to my room to the sound of more giggles. I told myself I wasn't going to get sensitive over stupid remarks, that I just didn't care. And I remembered Gerry from the Rehabilitation Unit. Yes, Gerry, it's hard not to care.

Policy at the hostel changed and males were accepted. The first I knew about it was when, wearing only my towelling robe, I was washing my hair in the communal washroom next to my bedroom. A young man came in who, without a word to me, proceeded to fill one of the other washbasins and begin to shave.

'I'm going to put two young men in your room,' Mrs Stroud announced later. I had visions of lying in bed in my small attic room with two snoring men in hammocks stretched across the room, but of course what she had in mind for me was less interesting than that. I was moved down a floor and into the smallest 'bedroom' imaginable, which had previously been a boxroom used for storing mops and brushes. All that would fit in it was a single bed with some storage space underneath. There was a one-bar electric fire in the only place there was room for it – high up on the wall, with a pull cord to switch it on and off. Of course there was no room for a wardrobe so I had to use one that was out in the corridor. Worst of all, there was no table on which I could write or type.

'Most of the others here need a desk or table because they're students. I didn't think you needed one,' Mrs Stroud said when I mentioned the subject.

'I'm studying for O levels so I've got essays to write and … and I do other writing besides. I need to use my typewriter.'

'Well, can't you sit on the bed and use it on your lap?'

Later that day I brought Vivian to see my new room.

'It's *awful!* It's so claustrophobic,' Vivian said. 'You ought to complain. You've lived here longer than some of the other residents and they've all got proper rooms.'

It didn't matter. I intended leaving anyhow and was scanning the paper each day in search of accommodation.

*　　　　　　*　　　　　　*

347

On a wintry Saturday morning, I moved into my 'furnished bed-sit, own kitchen, shared bathroom' on the first floor of a large, old, shabby terraced house. A nail was protruding from the wall above the fireplace and I had just the right thing to hang on it. I pulled out of my bag a joke notice I'd brought back from Somerset: a white card with fancy black lettering on it which read '**BLESS THIS MESS**'. How appropriate, I thought, as I hung it on the wall, chuckling to myself. I knew my bed-sit wasn't the kind of accommodation most people would get excited about but it was another step towards independence and, although the words 'dilapidated dump' would have been an apt description for it, nothing could take away my thrill of pleasure as I unpacked my bags and surveyed my new home.

CHAPTER THIRTY-ONE

MY SITUATION AT WORK improved dramatically when three new girls, Roz, Trish and Paula, started. Somehow we got talking and I soon got over my shyness with them (why this doesn't happen with everyone, I don't know). No more sitting alone in the canteen or at tea breaks. The work was still as boring, of course, but having people there whom I could laugh and talk with raised my daily portion of happiness to heights never before attained at work.

Paula and I got a month's extended leave from work to go travelling in Greece with Josie and Sarah, two of Paula's friends who were students at York University. As on the holiday in Somerset with Helen, I revelled in the joys of being alive, open to experiences again, and ... somehow, I couldn't quite believe this – still young!

I was happy, too, with my bed-sit despite all that was wrong with it. The sash window didn't fit into the framework properly. Wind, rain and snow came straight through, defying my attempts to block up the gaps with newspaper, cardboard or whatever I could find. When it rained heavily, a huge puddle would quickly form on the sill then spill over onto the floor so freely that I imagined the occupant of the bedsit below me having to sit watching TV with an umbrella. I survived bitterly cold winter nights by wearing thick woollen clothing over my pyjamas, a dressing-gown, and zipping myself up inside a sleeping bag with blankets piled on top.

I awoke with a start in the middle of my first night there. No, not the 'green light' dream again, I didn't have that now. My bed had collapsed! One of the legs had obviously been broken before and didn't fit properly, but a pile of books made the bed only slightly tilted. There was also a deceptively comfortable-looking rocking chair with a broken leg, and a broken buffet. The safest, and warmest, place to sit was on a tatty rug in front of the gas fire. Each time I opened the door from the inside of my room, the door knob came off in my hand – until I acquired the knack of turning the knob extremely slowly and carefully.

The previous occupant had made some attempt to turn the walls from a sickly mustard to a dreadful pink but had given up after half a wall. I kept meaning to try decorating the place myself but never got round to it. It wasn't worth buying decent curtains to get them saturated but I acquired some cheap ones from a jumble sale. The curtains that were up when I moved in didn't fit the windows, leaving about a three-inch gap when I drew them, so I took them down and used one at the door as a draught excluder and the other on the windowsill to catch and muffle the rain and snow.

The young man who lived in the attic room above me sometimes played his stereo late at night (like my brother used to) and I'd be trying to sleep with the annoying *thud, thud, thud* sound of the bass instruments. Once, at about three in the morning, he treated me to a loud rendering of 'Rule Britannia'. I sprang out of bed in a temper, grabbed my sweeping brush and, standing on the bed, banged on the ceiling with the brush handle. A shower of plaster fell onto my head, but he got the message and I got some peace. For weeks after this incident there was a welcome but eerie silence from above. Then one night I kept hearing a heavy thudding sound moving around his floor, which made my ceiling shudder and my light flicker. What the hell was he doing now? I found out later that he had a leg in plaster and was hopping across his room.

The light for the landing and stairway was on a timer to go out automatically. It was supposed to give you enough time to get up or down the stairs, but you'd need to be a prize-winning athlete to manage it. At night I always had to negotiate the last few stairs in the dark.

On the one occasion I went down into the basement of the house I stepped off the bottom of the stairs to find myself standing ankle-deep in dirty water.

'It's wicked of people to rent out houses that are in this state,' Vivian said.

I was very busy. There were lots of new things to learn, from getting just the right amount of soap in the machines at the launderette down the road to the realisation that man (or woman) cannot live by tinned food alone. My cookery skills were almost non-existent, so I bought the most basic cookery book I could find, and filled my bed-sit with weird and wonderful smells.

I was out most evenings. I had classes three nights a week, my aim being to get several O levels in the shortest possible time as I was keen to make up for my wasted years and get on to higher education. I was also enjoying myself at nights with my new friends from work, still visiting my old friends Jackie and Mandy occasionally (though they were both married now), plus seeing Helen and Vivian regularly. Vivian had recently graduated as a mature student and was shortly to take up a teaching post in London. I would miss her and our stimulating talks very much, but we planned to write often and meet when we could.

As time passed, my 'BLESS THIS MESS' notice started to look even more appropriate than when I first hung it on the wall. This won't do, I scolded myself, on arriving in late and tired one Friday night to trip over a pile of my belongings on the floor. I got up early the next morning to declare war on clutter. Where to begin? There was an overspill of books on the floor that wouldn't fit into the small bookcase which Ricky, Mandy's husband, had kindly made for me. I also had an assortment of papers and files that wouldn't fit into drawers. These were stuffed into four large carrier bags and left lying on the floor.

'I've got to stop hoarding things,' I told myself as I opened the first carrier bag, which contained two large ring binders with the notes made at evening classes the previous year. But I thought they might come in useful again as I intended to build on the basic knowledge gained and go into depth on whatever subjects most interested me.

The next carrier bag I looked inside contained lots of airmail letters from Mike. I reread a few of them and smiled sadly. I didn't love him, could never marry him, but he was a friend and neither of us seemed capable of breaking contact completely. I replaced the letters, unable to throw them out.

I delved into another carrier bag and pulled out some notebooks containing autobiographical poems written by Gerry. He had done a 'runner' before finishing his course at the unit and had given me his poems just before then. I reread them with a sigh and a tear. What they lacked in that indefinable quality called literary merit they made up for in their honest and poignant portrayal of the experience of being an outsider. I couldn't throw them out.

The fourth carrier bag contained my old diaries. Among these was the 1968 diary, which gave a painfully accurate description each day of my state of mind and circumstances as a troubled teenager, from the beginning of the year up to, and including, that fateful day of hospital admission in December. After that came the few extracts scribbled on toilet paper at the hospital and copied into my diary when home for Christmas. Later, in my 1969 diary, an entry written on a weekend leave: 'Slept all day'. After discharge from Thornville, a few more entries saying 'Slept all day'. Then blank pages. Nothing. It was as if I'd died. And in a way I had.

On rereading these diaries I was struck afresh with the way my treatment completely mismatched the problems for which I was supposedly being treated. It fuelled my anger, but I was so glad I'd written, and kept, these diaries, especially the 1968 one. Otherwise maybe I'd be wondering if I'd gone into hospital more 'sick' than I'd been aware of at the time or could now remember. Along with these diaries was my current journal and a folder containing papers on which I'd written my recent thoughts, mainly the questions about psychiatry that kept bouncing around in my head. This was part of my coming-to-terms writing. I had a lot more work to do before I could dispense with the contents of this bag.

So much for getting rid of the bags that cluttered my floor, but I did have more success in discarding some of the things which had accumulated in my drawers.

As I went through my hoard of belongings trying to sort things out, deciding where to put things, what to hold on to, what to discard, I knew my mind was undertaking a similar task. In my bed-sit, at work, out with friends, with my family, in the warmth and quiet of a library, amidst the noise and clamour of crowded places, at evening classes, tucked up inside my sleeping bag at night ... anywhere, everywhere, alone or with people, my inner struggle to come to terms continued, sometimes calmly and quietly, and sometimes in flames of anger or bursts of self-pity. Learning to deal constructively with my antagonism towards psychiatry was a lengthy and difficult process.

'What happened, Jean?' Jackie asked. 'Do you remember how not long before you first went to see a psychiatrist we were sitting here in this pub trying to understand how Christians can believe in a God of love sending people to hell to suffer for all eternity?'

I nodded, and smiled sadly. 'Yeah, I never did figure that one out.'

'When you told me you'd asked to see a psychiatrist, I was dying to find out what he'd say because I was just the same as you.'

'I remember how, when I told you I was going into hospital, we laughed at the thought of me "basket-making with the loonies", didn't we?' I stared into my lager.

Never again would I use an abusive term such as 'loonies' to describe those of us who, rightly or wrongly, receive psychiatric diagnoses. 'It seems an awfully long time ago, doesn't it?' I said, fiddling with a beer mat. 'Like something remembered from a previous life.'

'And then I saw you when you'd been in hospital a while, and I couldn't believe it. They'd turned you into a zombie! But before that, we were both just the same. I was as confused about religion and life as what you were. So what happened?'

'What happened was an attempt to cure my headache by chopping my head off,' I replied cynically. 'The psychiatric solution to misery. Oh, but pardon me, Doctor, I'd rather keep my head on. I do need it at times.'

'It doesn't make sense, Jean, treating you like they did.'

'No, and it doesn't make sense that I complied, and for so long. Who'll be the next to *volunteer* for the chopping block? Come this way, Jean, that's a good girl. God, I'm so angry with myself for allowing it to happen.'

'Don't blame yourself, Jean. How could you understand what was going on when you were so drugged? It's me who should've done summat when I saw you like that. Honestly, Jean, I feel so guilty for not trying to do anything.'

'Well, you'd better get off the guilt trip at once 'cos there was nowt you could've done. Remember how young we were, Jackie? Just a pair of silly teenagers.'

'We were both just the same,' Jackie said again. 'It could've happened to me.'

'How do I seem now?' I asked.

'Oh, like Sleeping Beauty who's at last woken up,' she said, with a grin. 'Seriously though, since stopping the tablets you're back to the old Jean I used to know. Thank goodness.'

'That's what Mandy says, but I'm not really,' I said, picking up my drink. 'The old Jean wasn't bitter and angry and cynical. I'll never be the same again.' I finished off my drink quickly. 'Still, at least I haven't ended up with two heads,' I added, smiling, in an attempt to avoid the self-pity trap.

'Don't kid yourself there, Jean,' Jackie said, giggling. 'A few more drinks and you might even have three.'

Wanting to make myself useful, I attended a course of evening classes aimed at giving a broad outline of different kinds of voluntary work. One evening the topic was 'Mental Health' and an invited speaker, a mental health professional, said that if hospitalisation, drugs or ECT was prescribed for a patient the role of the volunteer befriender could be to allay that patient's fears and encourage him or her to co-operate with the doctor.

It seemed to me both absurd and dangerous to believe that doctors were infallible. And if a wrong initial diagnosis was made, what chance was there of it being rectified once the person was in hospital for 'observation' where (as in my 'case') all the staff could observe was how a patient behaved while heavily drugged and in a certain kind of stressful (hospital) environment? Wouldn't the staff have preconceptions anyway about the 'already labelled' person? Once hospitalised, drugged and shocked, how could the effects of treatment be distinguished from whatever 'symptoms' were supposedly being treated? And how much did the doctors know about the causes of the thoughts, feelings or behaviour that supposedly needed treating? Can the complex range of human misery, with its opportunities for both damage and growth, really be legitimately reduced to crude diagnostic labels and theories about brain chemistry?

My brother once worked hard to annoy me so that he could record my angry reaction on a small, hidden tape recorder. Later, I heard him playing it back to laugh about with someone. I did sound upset. Weaker personality? Neurone transmitters not firing correctly? Poor coping responses? But only my voice was on the tape; the cause and context of my anger had been cut. How many psychiatrists are basing important treatment decisions on such a distorted, one-sided perspective?

All my questions raise further questions. Was (am?) I 'mentally ill' (whatever that means)? And, more importantly, because this applies whether or not I was 'mentally ill': what wisdom, morality, or even just basic common sense was there in the treatment I received?

Five wasted years. Years when I should have been living and learning and growing up. And what about others whose five years turns into fifty, sixty or seventy years, the ones who never make it back? How many of those are victims not of 'mental illness' but of psychiatry? We, who have survived the system intact enough to live and grow and write books about our experiences, are the lucky ones.

But what about the silenced? What about their stories?

AFTERWORD

'Doctors pour drugs of which they know little, to cure diseases of which they know less, into human beings of whom they know nothing.'

Voltaire

A LONG TIME HAS passed since Voltaire wrote that in the eighteenth century. A long time, too, has passed since the spring of 1974 when I swallowed my last psychiatric drug and 'FINISHED MY CONNECTIONS'. High Royds has been closed, along with the other large Victorian-built mental institutions. Does this reflect a radical change in attitudes, or is the 'change' only from one setting to another?

A lot is said, and written, about psychiatry by professional experts, but there is a crying need for more recipients and survivors of the psychiatric system to be heard. Although the User/Survivor movement, and others aware of the need for change, have brought about significant improvements in the past decade, there is still far to go. It is as imperative as ever to address the questions raised in this book, and for more of us to speak out about our experiences.

The most frightening thing about what happened to me is that most of it could still happen to a young person, or indeed anyone, today. I was a casualty of the narrow medical perspective of conventional psychiatry. With almost no knowledge of me or the context of my life, psychiatrists swiftly began treatment for what their training told them was an illness requiring brain-changing drugs and ECT. Over thirty years later, how has psychiatry changed? Psychiatry has arguably become even more biologically focused. An increasing number

357

of people experiencing misery due to relationships, employment, housing and other problems connected to life events are prescribed drugs such as Prozac to treat a perceived abnormality of brain neurotransmitters. ECT is still widely used.

I am not saying a medical framework of mental distress is always destructive as I do appreciate that some people find medication, and an understanding of their problems in terms of a diagnosis, helpful. But I, and many others, have learnt to our cost how limiting and damaging it can be to frame our experiences as symptoms of illness requiring physical treatments.

I read my case notes recently and have incorporated extracts from them into this book. What am I to make of these records? The diagnosis of schizophrenia was a complete surprise to me. I never had the so-called 'classic symptom' of hearing voices, nor did I experience psychotic delusions, a loosening of my grip on 'reality'. But a diagnosis of 'schizophrenia (simplex)' was, and still is, based on what are called 'negative symptoms of schizophrenia', such as social withdrawal, lethargy, blunted emotions. Ah, well ... add to these 'symptoms' those words of a mixed-up teenager: 'I do not know what I am' and 'I am confused with so many different ideas' including the religious ideas about 'heaven and hell', and there we have the evidence of 'thought disorder of bizarre in[sic] nature' – which all adds up to schizophrenia. Really?

How quickly, how easily, and on what flimsy 'evidence' diagnostic labels may be affixed and lives torn apart. Yet the serious flaws in the diagnostic process are still seemingly unacknowledged by those with unswerving belief in its scientific validity.

Today, as when I was a patient, the implications of being given such a diagnosis as schizophrenia can be extremely grave in terms of treatment decisions, employment prospects, self-concept, beliefs and attitudes of others towards the diagnosed person, stigmatisation, disempowerment, social isolation and misery; all in addition to whatever psychosocial problems there may have already been. Little wonder the prognosis for 'chronic schizophrenics' tends to be dismal (whether or not the diagnosis is correct).

So what about the problems which prompted me to seek psychiatric help in the first place? What about my shyness, family troubles, dissatisfaction with life, all that conflict and confusion about religion and the struggles to come to terms with the loss of my Christian faith? Whether psychiatric problems or 'growing pains', they were, of course, still there for me to deal with when I left the hospital and stopped taking drugs.

The shyness which caused a lot of sadness and misunderstanding didn't go away but it lessened. I made new friends, and I am still in touch with my 'old' close friends: Jackie, Mandy and Vivian.

Living away from my parents, I didn't feel a need to cut off all contact with them as my brother did. I am sure my parents (both dead now) loved me and they would not have knowingly done anything to harm me.

I left Ravens to work in the office of a social-work agency, while also doing voluntary work helping (I hope), mainly by empathic listening, those who were as unhappy and confused as I had once been. I then went on to study for a BA (Hons) degree in Combined Studies (mainly Literature and Psychology), slowly gaining the confidence to speak out in class discussions, and some of the positive relationships I formed with other mature students developed into strong friendships that endure today.

I still sometimes fear that ECT and psychiatric drugs damaged my brain, but at least some parts of it seem to be functioning well: I graduated with a First Class Honours degree.

My views on religion have not basically changed since I questioned, and lost, my beliefs in my teens. It would be pleasant to believe that we are watched over by a wise, caring God who will one day reveal to us what we cannot now understand, as in this poem:

> Not 'til the loom is silent
> And the shuttles cease to fly,
> Will God unroll the canvas
> And explain the reason why
> The dark threads are as needful
> In The Weaver's skilful hand
> As the threads of gold and silver
> In the pattern He has planned.

As a teenager I wanted badly to find a meaning, a purpose, a pattern, a God. To think as I started doing then, that there might be none of these things, was hard for me to take. Over the years I have learnt to live with ambiguities, uncertainty, the possibility of never knowing. But it seems that 'something' of my leanings towards spirituality never left me. Not completely. Words I read long ago from the poem above, written by Benjamin Malachi Franklin, have stayed in my mind, perhaps still inspiring me to search for the Divine Weaver who will one day explain the dark threads.

Writing this book has made me reflect upon what might have been, following on from what used to be: my dad stalking the town with a knife, my mum sleeping rough on some waste ground, my brother 'off his head' in 'every which way', and me written off as suffering from chronic schizophrenia. Bless this mess! And 'there but for fortune' I could have ended up a life-long psychiatric patient, emotionally crippled and a victim of tardive dyskinesia. Instead, my life became amazingly 'normal' and happy. Leaving home, finishing with psychiatry and getting off the drugs are not the answers for everyone but certainly enabled me to turn a depressing (untold) story into a story of triumph.

I began writing this book many years ago in my little room at the YWCA, sitting on my bed with my old, battered portable typewriter balanced on my knees. I continued it in my cold, draughty bed-sit and am finishing it on a PC in the warm, comfortable house where I live today with Ian, the man I love more than words can say. Memories and perceptions of past events are inevitably fallible but I have worked hard to recreate my experiences with scrupulous honesty, telling truths as I perceive them.

My work time is currently divided between writing, studying and working in mental health for an organisation affiliated to Mind. Years pass by much more quickly than they used to, so it seems I'll never find enough time to do all the things I want to do. How very different is my life now from existence in the bleak mental hospital world where time hung so heavily.

As I bring this book to a close, I am thinking about the patients I knew, wondering how many of them are still suffering. And I am remembering how one of them, Georgina, hugged me in tears on the day I left the hospital, saying that I would go away and forget all about them.

It's true that during the ups and downs of everyday living, memories of the hospital world and the sad plight of patients often recede. How could it be otherwise? I am awake and alive, and I've a wonderful husband with whom to share the joys and sorrows of living. So many things to do, places to go, people to meet, and always more new experiences, new things to learn; oh, still so much living to catch up on.

But, no, Georgina, I won't forget. I promise I'll never forget.

Narrow Margins

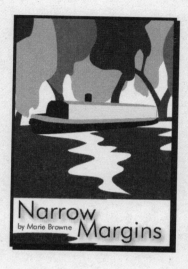

Faced with the loss of everything following the collapse of the Rover Group, Marie Browne moved her long-suffering husband Geoff, chaotic children and smelly, narcoleptic dog on to a houseboat in search of a less stressful, healthier, alternative way of life.

Narrow Margins – a laugh-out-loud book which proves that lean times can sometimes be a very positive thing.

ISBN 9781907016004   £7.99

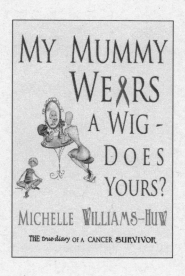

A true and heart-warming account of a journey through breast cancer.

A diagnosis of breast cancer made Michelle Williams-Huw, mother of two small boys, re-evaluate her life as she battled her demons to come to terms with the illness. *My Mummy Wears A Wig* is poignant, sad, revelatory and deliciously funny. Readers will be riveted by her honesty and enchanted as, having hit bottom, she falls in love with life (and her husband) all over again.

ISBN 9781906125110   £7.99

No Legs To Dance On
A Thalidomide survivor's story

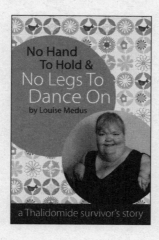

Louise was born Louise Mason, a victim of the devastating drug Thalidomide. Born without arms and legs, she is the daughter of David Mason, who single-handedly held out against the drug company, the legal establishment and all the other parents of Thalidomide victims in the high-profile fight for proper compensation for the victims. As she was photographed with her family and appeared on television meeting celebrities during the battle, few people realised that she did not live with her wealthy parents and three siblings at their spacious North London home but was being brought up in an institution, Chailey Heritage in Sussex. In fact, Louise had never gone home from hospital and, for the first five weeks of her life, her mother didn't even see her.

ISBN 9781906373573 £9.99

Diary of a Diet
- The Little Book of Big

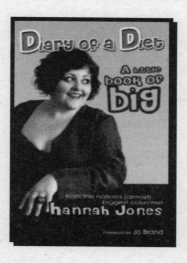

The book that eats the Size Zero debate for breakfast and coughs it back up with a side of comedy carbs, features the ordered ramblings of outsized and outspoken newspaper columnist Hannah Jones. Her diary will find resonance with all women, whatever their shape or size, who've felt pressure to weigh out their self-esteem along with their chips. It's a sharp, witty and heartfelt study on living life in the fat - oops, sorry! - fast lane to self-acceptance.

Diary of a Diet is about Hannah Jones' ongoing struggle to commit to get fit, stick to a sensible eating plan or think, once and for all, that she's simply fabulous just the way she is right now.

ISBN 9781906125042   £6.99

Listening In

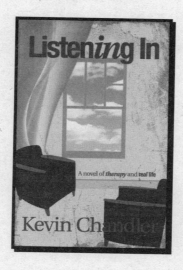

A novel of therapy and real life which allows the reader to eavesdrop behind the closed door of the therapy room

The therapist and prostitute have more in common than you think. Both charge by the hour for intimate services that most people find for free within a personal relationship, and both conceal their personal selves behind their professional personas and strict rules of engagement

Kevin Chandler is a private therapist, specialising in relationship, marital, and sexual therapy, based in Yorkshire. He has trained many Relate counsellors during his career. *Listening In* is his first novel.

ISBN 9781906373658   £7.99

For more information about Accent Press
titles please visit

www.accentpress.co.uk